T0262667

Anxiety Disorders

Anxiety Disorders

Edited by **Peter Garner**

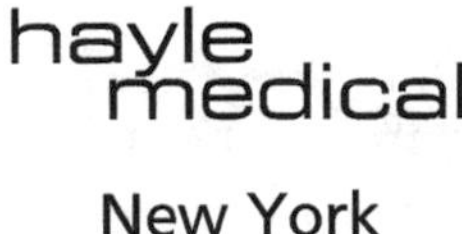

New York

Published by Hayle Medical,
30 West, 37th Street, Suite 612,
New York, NY 10018, USA
www.haylemedical.com

Anxiety Disorders
Edited by Peter Garner

International Standard Book Number: 978-1-63241-047-4 (Hardback)

Printed in the United States of America.

Contents

Preface

It is often said that books are a boon to humankind. They document every progress and pass on the knowledge from one generation to the other. They play a crucial role in our lives. Thus I was both excited and nervous while editing this book. I was pleased by the thought of being able to make a mark but I was also nervous to do it right because the future of students depends upon it. Hence, I took a few months to research further into the discipline, revise my knowledge and also explore some more aspects. Post this process, I begun with the editing of this book.

This book consists of contributions made by several clinical psychiatrists from across the globe, aimed at developing general research regarding anxiety and applying it in clinical contexts. Up-to-date information regarding the field has been presented in this book, outlining the clinical pitfalls. It encompasses two sections on basic matters about anxiety and fundamental research matters on particular aspects of anxiety.

I thank my publisher with all my heart for considering me worthy of this unparalleled opportunity and for showing unwavering faith in my skills. I would also like to thank the editorial team who worked closely with me at every step and contributed immensely towards the successful completion of this book. Last but not the least, I wish to thank my friends and colleagues for their support.

Editor

Section 1

General Issues

Chapter 1

Anxiety: An Adaptive Emotion

Ana G. Gutiérrez-García and Carlos M. Contreras

Additional information is available at the end of the chapter

1. Introduction

Anxiety as an adaptive response is a natural emotion that occurs in response to danger and prepares an organism to cope with the environment, playing a critical role in its survival. Among the components of anxiety, the expression of fear may inform other members of the group about the presence of imminent danger (i.e., an alarm cue). The environment is perceived by a filtering process that involves sensorial receptors. While coping with a stressful situation, an individual may simultaneously emit vocalizations, perform movements to escape, freeze, and deliver to the environment chemicals called alarm pheromones. These cues are recognized by the receptor-individual by specific sensory systems located in the legs and antennae in insects and olfactory sensorial systems in other organisms. In mammals, the sensorial information is integrated by anatomical and functional pathways, with the participation of structures related to emotional memory, namely deep temporal lobe structures. Some stimuli are perceived as relevant when they contain relevant meaning according to previous experience and learning. The participation of ventral striatum and prefrontal cortex connections then leads to the selection of an adequate strategy for survival. The perception of these cues by other individuals in the group establishes intraspecies communication and causes striking behavioral responses in the receptor subject, namely anxiety, but the consequence is likely different. While the emitting subject may be in an emergency situation that is perhaps devoid of a solution, the receptor subject may have the chance to cope with the dangerous situation by employing efficacious strategies, depending on previous experience. The aim of this chapter is to review the participation of such anatomical pathways, their neurotransmission systems, and the resulting behavioral patterns.

2. Expression of fear and anxiety as emotions

Emotions are transient events generated in response to some stimuli that produce arousal reactions and changes in motor behavior, subjective feelings, and subsequent changes in behavior [15]. Thus, emotions are cognitive and somatic reactions, with a short duration, to specific environmental stimuli [7]. In the case of an emergency situation, emotions give way to strategies that allow the survival of the individual and, therefore, the species. Emotional processes are crucial for the control of human behavior [15], and a failure in the management of emotions is a common denominator of a wide range of psychiatric disorders [22].

In broad terms, emotions are considered to have two dimensions. The first dimension is equilibrium, in which emotional states range from positive (i.e., happy or safe) to negative (i.e., fear or anger). The consequent behavioral responses depend on emotional states. For example, in a positive emotional state, there is a tendency to approach the stimuli, whereas negative emotional states are associated with aversion, defense, escape, and avoidance. The second dimension is arousal. Both positive and negative emotional states may vary from a relatively quiet attitude to high levels of restlessness [54; 53]. Examples include freezing in a passive attitude or escaping in more proactive coping patterns [20]. Emotions play a role in the daily lives of individuals, enabling them to cope with everyday situations.

Fear is a part of the anxiety syndrome. It consists of a feeling of agitation caused by the presence of imminent danger and may be considered a protective emotion. From an evolutionary point of view, however, its expression is very similar to anxiety as an adaptive emotion. An exception may be posttraumatic stress, an anxiety disorder in which fear is present even in the absence of the stimulus that elicited the original state of anxiety [100]. Notably, fear can be conditioned by various stimuli, and its study from different methodological perspectives has allowed a better comprehension of the underlying neurobiological processes of anxiety.

3. Is anxiety a disease or an adaptive response?

Anxiety comprises two related concepts. First, it is a disease. Second, it is an adaptive response. As a disease, anxiety is a highly disabling pathological condition, involving cognitive, emotional, and physiological disturbances. Its main symptoms include restlessness, increased alertness, motor tension, and increased autonomic activity [2]. In the long-term, the deleterious effects of anxiety on personal capabilities represents a considerable mental health problem. Generalized anxiety disorder is frequently associated with other pathologies, but it may constitute the only symptom in several manifestations, including panic disorder, posttraumatic stress disorder, and obsessive compulsive disorder [2]. It is one of the most common psychiatric disorders, affecting approximately 28% of the general population [49]. In México, as in other countries, it occurs more often in women than in men [64]. Typically, the symptoms last a long time, even when the stimulus has disappeared [100].

Adaptive anxiety may be considered a useful emotion that leads to survival strategies [4]. In this sense, anxiety is a normal emotion that occurs when an individual copes with a potentially dangerous situation, constituting a mechanism for alertness or alarm [41]. In this case, the symptoms of anxiety, which are identical to the pathological condition, disappear once the stressful stimulus disappears. Meanwhile, in most cases, it leads to coping with the emergency situation. As the best strategy is chosen, the probability of ensuring survival increases.

One of the main differences between the two kinds of anxiety is the contingency of the response to the stimulus. Otherwise, pathological anxiety induces positive feedback, in which anxiety generates more anxiety [75] and, notably, spreads to other individuals in the group [88; 24]. The combination of feedback and the spread of anxiety can lead to a collective panic reaction that involves those individuals who surrounded the first individual who experienced anxiety [89], often with fatal results [74; 62]. One very special case is related to caregivers. Observing a state of anxiety that leads to deteriorated social functioning and health is common in caregivers, with undesirable effects in both the caregiver and patient [94]. Therefore, anxiety may be both a disease and an adaptive response that involves shared processes and in some cases may inclusively consist of a continuum.

4. Anxiety is contagious

In the case of anxiety as an adaptive emotion that leads to survival strategies, the spread of anxiety to other individuals in the group may offer warning signs that allow for the protection of other individuals and consequently the group and ultimately the species [6].

Generally, all stimuli derived from the environment initially undergo a sensorial filtering process in sensorial receptors, beginning with parareceptors [8], reaching synaptic relays, and leading to an integrative process that involves anatomical structures related to emotional memory [43], in which comparisons are made with older elements of memory [92]. As the stimulus inputs reach the striatum and cortical structures [43], a selection of the adequate survival strategy is often reached [34]. In turn, connections with motor areas and motoneurons activates skeletal muscles [43], and a motoric response may be observed. Laboratory animals subjected to a stressful situation (e.g., odors from a predator) will emit only a few responses—attacking, freezing, or escaping—no more and no less.

One important aspect is the meaning of the stimuli. Only a portion of all environmental stimuli is perceived as relevant when it contains a specific meaning according to previous experience. Any of these stimuli may potentially contain relevant environmental information, but its relevance arises when it is properly interpreted. The contrast between the present stimuli and previous experience allows predictions to be made about the real presence or absence of danger and selecting the correct coping response [34; 63]. An intriguing aspect is that most studies of the neural and behavioral framework of these types of motor responses have been performed in laboratory animals (i.e., animals that were completely naive of predators before the test). However, some studies in naturally free animals have found similar results [19; 90]. The interpretation is that a neural framework adapted by natural selection is able to respond in some effective way, even in the absence of any previous experience. Therefore, the neural framework allows an initial response to any dangerous situation in the environment, yielding necessarily useful strategies for survival. Choosing the best strategy to cope with such situations depends on experience (i.e., learning).

5. Communication and anxiety

During natural selection and evolution, several organisms have developed strategies that allow different but complementary forms of communication between individuals of the same species. Thus, animal communication includes the emission and reception of signals delivered in the environment, usually following some specific code. Moreover, communication also includes behaviors in the receptor-individual. Success in the detection of cues includes a series of processes that consist of emission of the cue, reception by other individuals, encoding, transmission, and decoding [26].

Notably, special situations, such as emergency situations, involve most of the sensorial systems. A primitive form of communication is body language. In this case, environmental information is detected by the visual system. Insects frequently apparently dance while performing stereotyped movements [33] that apparently carry a message whose meaning is not yet fully understood.

The auditory system is involved in the most complex of these forms of communication. A symbolic language that contains a characteristic syntactic structure is apparently peculiar to the human species [79]. In a more primitive form, nonsyntactic and perhaps only symbolic language is observed in other species [6]. In fact, animal vocalizations are devoid of semantic content (i.e., meaning) but posses some semiotic context that contains symbolic value [16]. The signals generated by animals are used for communication and consist of signs that become messages that are capable of influencing the behavior of other individuals who are also able to respond with species-typical signals by distinguishing its semiotic content. For example, most ultrasonic vocalizations of animals, including rats, are true semiotic signs and represent a useful signal within a communication system [63]. Most of these semiotic signals may represent warning cues that seemingly produce some anxiety responses in other individuals of the same species.

Among the signaling systems, chemical cues that consist of pheromones [48] can cause striking behavioral responses, including anxiety [31; 32], when perceived by other individuals of the group. The opposite is also true. Some pheromones consist of cues that indicate the existence of a safe environment [47; 103] by informing other individuals of the same species about the absence of danger or presence of food. In both cases, an emitting-individual releases substances to the environment that are recognized by the receptor-individual by specific sensory systems located, for example, in the legs and antennae in insects [81] or olfactory sensory system in other organisms, including mammals [58]. Figure 1.

6. Neuroanatomical modeling of emotions

Emotional memory allows an individual to recognize signs from the environment and compare them with past experience as an element of judgment to efficaciously respond to the environment by choosing the best coping strategy [14]. During the first half of the 20th century, researchers were interested in the brain mechanisms of emotional behavior [57], and the original concept of the "limbic system" was gradually abandoned. Instead, the very simple, initial anatomical concept (i.e., hippocampus, one thalamic nuclei, mammillary bodies, and cingulum) was enriched by the inclusion of other deep temporal lobe structures, such as the amygdaloid complex [57], so-called mesolimbic structures [73], and prefrontal and orbitofrontal cortices [100]. All of these anatomical regions share similar neurotransmission systems, namely serotonin, norepinephrine, dopamine, and γ-aminobutyric acid (GABA), among others.

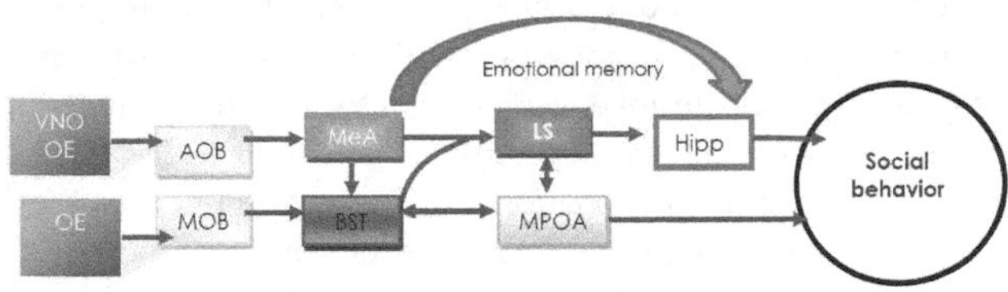

Figure 1. Social recognition and olfactory pathways in rodents. Abbrev. VNO, vomeronasal organ; OE, olfactory epithelium; AOB, accessory olfactory bulb; MOB, main olfactory bulb; MeA, medial amygdala; BST, bed nucleus of the stria terminalis; LS, lateral septal nucleus; MPOA, medial preoptic area; Hipp, hippocampus.

Some alterations in the serotonergic system are associated with psychiatric disorders, such as depression and schizophrenia [87]. Serotonin (5-hydroxytryptamine [5-HT]) is located primarily in the gastrointestinal tract, but it is also detectable in the central nervous system [29] in areas that are functionally related to many behavioral processes. Its main reservoir in the brain is the dorsal raphe nucleus [40; 78], which, among other projections, sends efferent fibers to several structures related to emotional processing, such as the septum, thalamus, amygdaloid complex, nucleus accumbens, hippocampus, and prefrontal cortex [29; 78]. Although a controversial issue [87], an increase of 5-HT in the synaptic cleft exerts anxiolytic effects in animal models of anxiety, such as the social interaction test, light-dark test, Vogel conflict test, Geller-Seifter conflict test, and ultrasonic vocalizations [10, 65], which have been confirmed by many clinical studies [60].

Norepinephrine is related to many functions, such as attention, the regulation of stress, fear, memory, sleep, and wakefulness [27]. It is synthesized in a small group of cells located in the locus coeruleus that sends efferent fibers parallel to those of 5-HT [40; 27]. Norepinephrine is involved in the secretion of corticotrophin-releasing factor, which stimulates the production of adrenocorticotropic hormone that, in turn, releases corticosterone in the adrenal glands, which is responsible of the metabolic response to stress [100; 67; i.e. an inseparable component of anxiety]. Anxiety is directly related to increased activity of locus coeruleus neurons. Drugs that increase noradrenergic activity also increase anxiety, and drugs that reduce noradrenergic activity reduce anxiety [40, 27]. Limbic and cortical regions innervated by the locus coeruleus are those that are thought to be involved in the elaboration of adaptive responses to stress, such as the typical scheme seen in fearful behavior in cats [1].

γ-Aminobutyric acid is a neurotransmitter distributed throughout the central nervous system and the quintessential inhibitory neurotransmitter [72]. Modulation of the GABAergic system at its receptors [5] is linked to the neurobiological mechanisms that regulate anxiety [72; 70; 86]. Most drugs with affinity for the $GABA_A$ receptor produce anxiolysis and sedation [96]. These receptors are detectable in the cerebral cortex, amygdala, hippocampus, and striatum [40], providing the physiological basis for the therapeutic action of anxiolytics [72], including gonadal steroids and neurosteroids [25; 12; 61].

Mesolimbic dopamine is found in the ventral tegmental area and involved in the control of cognition and affect [46]. Dopamine innervation of the medial prefrontal cortex appears to be particularly involved in mild and brief stress processing [21]. In turn, the prefrontal cortex plays a role in working memory, in addition to other brain areas, such as the hippocampus. A critical range of dopamine turnover is necessary to keep the working memory system active and ready for optimal cognitive functioning [42], a situation that is impaired in situations of extreme stress [3]. In summary, the dopamine system is important for general emotional responses, selective information processing, hedonic impact, and reward learning. In a broader sense, dopamine is important for reactivity to perturbations in the environment, which is essential for the ability (or failure) to cope with the environment [73; 99].

Multiple neurotransmission systems participate in the processing of anxiety and coping with the environment. Many other neurotransmitters are involved in the regulation of anxiety, including neuropeptides [91], polypeptides [95], and amino acids [104]. Nonetheless, a common denominator is that almost all of these neurotransmitters are located within the anatomical substrate of emotional memory [99], namely the amygdala complex [83].

The amygdala is composed of many functionally heterogeneous nuclei [56]. The lateral and central nuclei of the amygdala mediate the acquisition and expression of reactive defensive behaviors [59; 69], and the basal nucleus plays a key role in fear expression [38]. The basal amygdala nucleus, together with the lateral nucleus and accessory basal nucleus, integrate the basolateral amygdala [84]. As a whole, an increase in the neuronal firing rate of the basolateral amygdala has been related to fear [76], anxiety [101], emotional learning [17], and Pavlovian conditioning [28]. The basal amygdala nucleus appears to mediate fear-motivated reactions [55] but not conditioned auditory fear responses, such as freezing [69]. The central nucleus of the amygdala projects to various brain structures via the stria terminalis and ventral amygdalofugal pathway. The anatomical circuit responsible for the startle reflex begins in auditory pathways and reaches the central amygdala nucleus [18]. Pathways from the amygdala to lateral hypothalamus are related to peripheral sympathetic responses to stress [45]. Early findings reported that electrical stimulation of the amygdala in cats produced peripheral signs of autonomic hyperactivity and fear-related behavior, commonly seen when the animal attacks or is being attacked [39]. Electrical stimulation of the amygdala in human subjects also produces signs and symptoms of fear and anxiety, namely increased heart rate, blood pressure, and muscle tension, accompanied by subjective sensations of fear and anxiety [9] and an increase in plasma catecholamines [30]. Important reciprocal connections also exist between cortical association areas, the thalamus, and the amygdala, which may account for fear responses [82]. These findings demonstrate that the amygdala plays an important role in conditioned fear and the modulation of peripheral stress responses.

7. Fear and anxiety as a consequence of natural selection

The relationship between mother and child is essential for the survival and normal development of infants [71; 85]. Maternal odors attract and guide neonates to the maternal breast [98]. The role of mothers is to provide a source of nutrition for their offspring, but also to protect them from predators [80; 71]. Maternal odors produce signs of calm. Kittens, pups, and human babies exhibit increased agitation and vocalizations when placed in an unfamiliar environment, but when they return to their nest or stay in close proximity to their mother, they calm down [66; 85]. Amniotic fluid olfaction reduces crying in human babies when they are separated from their mothers [97]. Recently, we analyzed human amniotic fluid, colostrum, and breast milk. Eight fatty acids were consistently found in measurable amounts in these three biological fluids. Both amniotic fluid and a mixture of its fatty acids acted as feeding cues, leading to appetitive behavior [11]. Moreover, both amniotic fluid and a mixture of its fatty acids exerted anxiolytic effects in animal models of anxiety [13]. These findings indicate that a system of protection against anxiety is present during intrauterine life, at least in mammals, suggesting a process of natural selection in which an individual is protected from extreme anxiety, even before birth.

With regard to the opposite process, alarm cues (i.e., pheromones) are released by an animal in threatening situations, informing members of the same species about the presence of danger (e.g., the proximity of a predator; 36). The responses of conspecifics to alarm pheromones include fear, autonomic responses, and freezing [51], increased awareness [35], defensive behavior [52], and an increase in anxiety-like behavior (32; 44; i.e., some behaviors mediated by deep temporal lobe structures). A single exposure to predator odors (i.e., 2,3,5-trimethyl-3-tiazoline) contained in fox feces and cats increased *c-fos* expression in the lateral septal nucleus and central amygdala [19; 90], among other structures. An arterial spin labeling-based functional magnetic resonance imaging study found that neuronal activity increased in the dorsal periaqueductal gray, superior colliculus, and medial thalamus during alarm pheromone exposure [50]. Exposure to odors from potential predators also elicited fast waves in the dentate gyrus [37] and enhanced long-term potentiation in the dentate gyrus [23]. Both the main and accessory olfactory systems are responsive to 2-heptanone [102]. The medial amygdala nucleus receives indirect inputs from the main olfactory system from the piriform cortex, periamygdaloid cortex, and cortical amygdala nucleus and direct inputs from the accessory olfactory system [92]. The hippocampus also receives odor information from both olfactory systems through entorhinal cortex connections [77]. Herein, neurons from medial and cortical amygdala nuclei are activated in the presence of alarm pheromones [52], and the medial amygdala is involved in the neuronal circuitry associated with memory formation related to odors derived from predators, further leading to the expression of unconditioned and conditioned fear behavior [68; 93]. Figure 2.

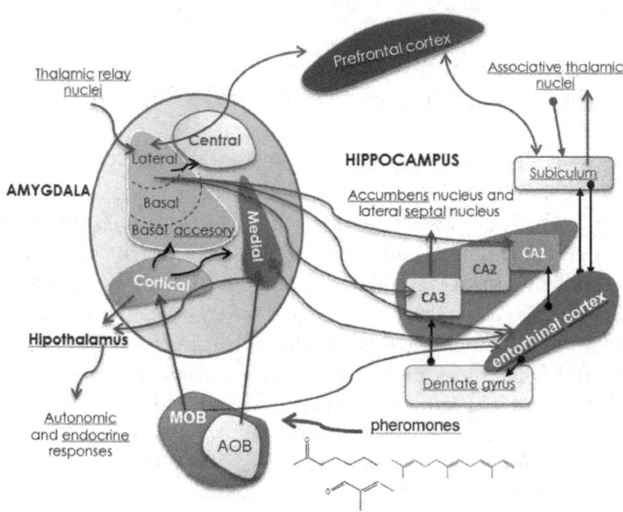

Figure 2. Anatomical representation of emotional memory circuit. Connections between amygdala and hippocampus, modulate the use of memories related to sensorial stimuli. Abbrev.: AOB, accessory olfactory bulb, MOB, main olfactory bulb.

8. Conclusions

Most of the known responses to alarm cues have come from studies in laboratory animals that reproduce and feed under relatively comfortable conditions. They live inside very well controlled facilities, distant from predators and dangerous situations. One may reconsider the concept of the rhinencephalon, an almost forgotten anatomical entity that involves brain structures (Figure 3) related to emotional memory and is present in mammals, reptiles, and birds. The rhinencephalon, at least as a concept, contains one of the primitive sources of capturing information from the environment—the olfactory system. The concept is completed by connections of this sensorial system with deep temporal lobe structures (i.e., emotional memory-related structures). Therefore, the existence of the rhinencephalon in many species suggests that the integration of anxiety responses is a broad, essential characteristic determined by natural selection. In such a case, anxiety as an adaptive response is common to species with a centralized nervous system. Anxiety as an adaptive response is also naturally contained in the brain, and it is expressed even before the organism learns the most efficacious behavioral response.

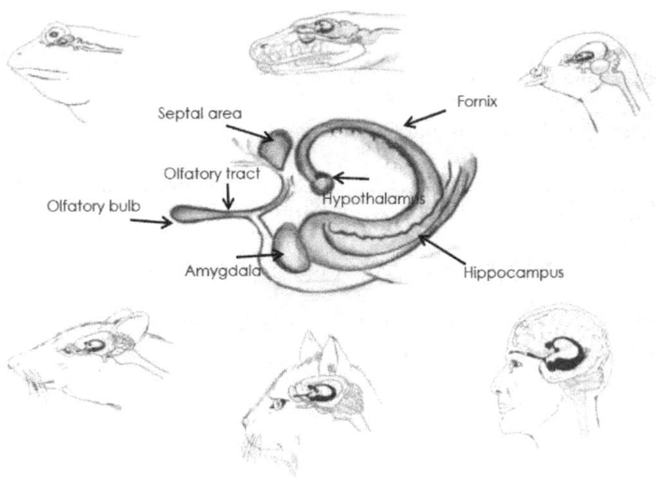

Figure 3. Squematic representation of rhinencephalon in several species. Since on evolution point of view (shaded area), rhinencephalon represents as integrative and primitive framework present in the central nervous system, integrating emotions escential for survivance, such as fear and anxiety.

Nature protects the mother and fetus during intrauterine development, in which the development of the fetus occurs in an environment that protects it from anxiety. Especially in mammals, early learning acquired through maternal-infant interactions during the first phase of life and subsequent learning acquired through interactions with dominant members of a given group allow the individual to learn to select the most effective survival strategy, with the participation of prefrontal brain structures.

Consequently, two processes occur. One process depends on the neural framework that will respond even in the absence of any previous experience. The other process is a consequence of learning. Working together, the outcome is the utility of anxiety as an adaptive reaction that contributes to the survival of the species.

Acknowledgements

The authors thank Michael Arends for revising and editing the English of this manuscript. The preparation of this chapter was partially supported by grants from the Consejo Nacional de Ciencia y Tecnología, México (CONACyT: CB-2006-1, 61741), Universidad Nacional

Autónoma de México (UNAM: DGAPA-PAPIIT IN211111-3), and Sistema Nacional de Investigadores (SNI, Exp. AGG-32755 and CMC-754).

Author details

Ana G. Gutiérrez-García[1,2] and Carlos M. Contreras[1,3*]

*Address all correspondence to: ccontreras@uv.mx

1 Laboratorio de Neurofarmacología, Instituto de Neuroetología, Universidad Veracruzana, Xalapa, Veracruz, México

2 Facultad de Psicología, Universidad Veracruzana, Xalapa, Veracruz, México

3 Unidad Periférica Xalapa, Instituto de Investigaciones Biomédicas, Universidad Nacional Autónoma de México, Xalapa, Veracruz, México

References

[1] Abercrombie, E. D, & Jacobs, B. L. (1987). Microinjected clonidine inhibits noradrenergic neurons of the locus coeruleus in freely moving cats. *Neurosci Lett*, 76(2), 203-208.

[2] American Psychiatric Association . (2000). Diagnostic and statistical manual of mental disorders, 4th edition. Washington, DC: American Psychiatric Association.

[3] Arnsten, A. F. (2000). Stress impairs prefrontal cortical function in rats and monkeys: role of dopamine D1 and norepinephrine α-1 receptor mechanisms. *Prog Brain Res*, 126, 183-192.

[4] Becerra-garcía, A. M, Madalena, A. C, Estanislau, C, Rodríguez-rico, J. L, & Dias, H. (2007). Ansiedad y miedo: su valor adaptativo y maladaptaciones. *Rev Latinoamericana Psicol*, 39(1), 75-81.

[5] Bormann, J. (2000). The "ABC" of GABA receptors. *Trends Pharmacol Sci*, 21(1), 16-19.

[6] Brudzynski, S. M. (2005). Principles of rat communication: quantitative parameters of ultrasonic calls in rats. *Behav Genet*, 35(1), 85-92.

[7] Buchanan, T. W. (2007). Retrieval of emotional memories. *Psychol Bull*, 133(5), 761-779.

[8] Carlson, N. R. (2001). Physiology and Behavior. 7th edition. Boston: Allyn and Bacon.

[9] Chapman, D. W. (1954). Anxiety heart disease. *Med Bull US Army Eur*, 11(9), 211-216.

[10] Clement, Y, & Chapouthier, G. (1998). Biological bases of anxiety. *Neurosci Biobehav Rev*, 22(5), 623-633.

[11] Contreras, C. M, Gutiérrez-García, A. G, Mendoza-López, M. R, Rodríguez-Landa, J. F, Bernal-Morales, B, & Díaz-Marte, C. (2012). Amniotic fluid elicits appetitive responses in human newborns: fatty acids and appetitive responses. *Dev Psychobiol*, in press.

[12] Contreras, C. M, Molina, M, Saavedra, M, & Martínez-Mota, L. (2000). Lateral septal neuronal firing increases during proestrus-estrus in the rat. *Physiol Behav*, 68, 279-284.

[13] Contreras, C. M, Rodríguez-Landa, J. F, Gutiérrez-García, A. G, Mendoza-López, M. R, García-Ríos, R. I, & Cueto-Escobedo, J. (2011). Anxiolytic-like effects of human amniotic fluid and its fatty acids in Wistar rats. *Behav Pharmacol*, 22, 655-662.

[14] Contreras, C. M, & Gutiérrez-García, A. G. (2010). Emotional memory and chemical communication. In: Benítez-King, G. & Cisneros-Berlanga, C. (eds)., *The neurobiological sciences applied to psychiatry: from genes, proteins, and neurotransmitters to behavior*, 171-188, Kerala: Research Signpost.

[15] Critchley, H. (2003). Emotion and its disorders. *Br Med Bull*, 65, 35-47.

[16] Danesi, M. (1993). Messages and meanings: an introduction to semiotics. Toronto: Canadian Scholars' Press.

[17] Davis, M, & Whalen, P. J. (2001). The amygdala: vigilance and emotion. *Mol Psychiatry*, 6, 13-34.

[18] Davis, M. (1992). The role of the amygdala in fear and anxiety. *Annu Rev Neurosci*, 15, 353-375.

[19] Day, H. E, Masini, C. V, & Campeau, S. (2004). The pattern of brain c-fos mRNA induced by a component of fox odor, 2,5-dihydro-2,4,5 trimethylthiazoline (TMT), in rats, suggests both systemic and processive stress characteristics. *Brain Res*, 1025(1-2), 139-151.

[20] De-Boer, S. F, & Koolhaas, J. M. (2003). Defensive buyring in rodents: ethology, neurobiology and psychopharmacology. *Eur J Pharmacol*, 463(1-3), 145-161.

[21] Deutch, A. Y, & Roth, R. H. (1990). The determinants of stress-induced activation of the prefrontal cortical dopamine system. *Prog Brain Res*, 85, 367-402.

[22] Dolan, R. J. (2002). Emotion, cognition, and behavior. *Science*, 298(5596), 1191-1194.

[23] Dringenberg, H. C, Oliveira, D, & Habib, D. (2008). Predator (cat hair)-induced enhancement of hippocampal long-term potentiation in rats: involvement of acetylcholine. *Learn Mem*, 15(3), 112-116.

[24] Elizarrarás-Rivas, J, Vargas-Mendoza, J. E, Mayoral-García, M, Matadamas-Zarate, C, Elizarrarás-Cruz, A, Taylor, M, & Agho, K. (2010). Psychological response of family

members of patients hospitalised for influenza A/H1N1 in Oaxaca, Mexico. *BMC Psychiatry*, 10, 104.

[25] Fernández-Guasti, A, Martínez-Mota, L, Estrada-Camarena, E, Contreras, C. M, & López-Ruvalcava, C. (1999). Chronic treatment with desipramine induces an estrous cycle-dependent anxiolytic-like action in the burying behavior, but not in the elevated plus-maze test. *Pharmacol Biochem Behav*, 63, 13-20.

[26] Green, S, & Marler, P. (1979). The analysis of animal communication. In: Marler, P. & Vandenbergh, J.G. (eds)., *Social behavior and communication (series title: Handbook of behavioral neurobiology*,, 3, 73-158, New York: Plenum Press.

[27] Goddard, A. W, Ball, S. G, Martinez, J, Robinson, M. J, Yang, C. R, Russell, J. M, & Shekhar, A. (2010). Current perspectives of the roles of the central norepinephrine system in anxiety and depression. *Depress Anxiety*, 27(4), 339-350.

[28] Grace, A. A, & Rosenkranz, J. A. (2002). Regulation of conditioned responses of basolateral amygdala neurons. *Physiol Behav*, 77, 489-493.

[29] Grahame-Smith, D. G. (1988). Serotonine (5-hydroxytrypatmine, 5-HT). *Q J Med*, 67(3), 459-466.

[30] Gunne, L. M, & Reis, D. J. (1963). Changes in brain catecholamines associated with electrical stimulation of amygdaloid nucleus. *Life Sci*, 11, 804-809.

[31] Gutiérrez-García, A. G, & Contreras, C. M. (2002). Algunos aspectos etológicos de la comunicación química en ratas y ratones de laboratorio. *Rev Bioméd*, 13, 189-209.

[32] Gutiérrez-García, A. G, Contreras, C. M, Mendoza-López, M. R, Cruz-Sánchez, S, García-Barradas, O, Rodríguez-Landa, J. F, & Bernal-Morales, B. (2006). A single session of emotional stress produces anxiety in Wistar rats. *Behav Brain Res*, 167(1), 30-35.

[33] Hammer, M, & Menzel, R. (1995). Learning and memory in the honeybee. *J Neurosci*, 15(3 Pt 1), 1617 -30 .

[34] Hasson, O. (1994). Cheating signals. *J Theor Biol*, 167, 223-238.

[35] Hauser, R, Marczak, M, Karaszewski, B, Wiergowski, M, Kaliszan, M, Penkowski, M, Kernbach-Wighton, G, Jankowski, Z, & Namiesnik, J. (2008). A preliminary study for identifying olfactory markers for fear in the rat. *Lab Anim*, 37, 76-80.

[36] Hauser, R, Wiergowski, M, Kaliszan, M, Gos, T, Kernbach-Wighton, G, Studniarek, M, Jankowski, Z, & Namiesnik, J. (2011). Olfactory and tissue markers of fear in mammals including humans. *Med Hypotheses*, 77, 1062-1067.

[37] Heale, V. R, Vanderwolf, C. H, & Kavaliers, M. (1994). Components of weasel and fox odors elicit fast wave bursts in the dentate gyrus of rats. *Behav Brain Res*, 63(2), 159-165.

[38] Herry, C, Ciocchi, S, Senn, V, Demmou, L, Muller, C, & Lüthi, A. (2008). Switching on and off fear by distinct neuronal circuits. *Nature*, 454, 600-606.

[39] Hilton, S. M, & Zbrozyna, A. W. (1963). Amygdaloid region for defense reactions and its efferent pathway to the brain stem. *J Physiol*, 165, 160-173.

[40] Hoehn-saric, R. (1982). Neurotransmitters in anxiety. *Arch Gen Psychiatry*, 39(6), 735-742.

[41] Hommer, D. W, Skolnick, P, & Paul, S. M. (1987). The benzodiazepine/GABA receptor complex and anxiety. In Meltzer, H.Y. (ed)., *Psychopharmacology: the third generation of progress*, 977-983, New York: Raven Press.

[42] Horger, B. A, & Roth, R. H. (1996). The role of mesoprefontal dopamine neurons in stress. *Crit Rev Neurobiol*, 10, 395-418.

[43] Hughes, M. (2004). Olfaction, emotion and the amygdala: arousal-dependent modulation of long-term autobiographical memory and its association with olfaction: beginning to unravel the Proust phenomenon? *Premier J Undergraduate Publ Neurosci*, 1(1), 1-58.

[44] Inagaki, H, Kiyokawa, Y, Kikusui, T, Takeuchi, Y, & Mori, Y. (2008). Enhancement of the acoustic startle reflex by an alarm pheromone in male rats. *Physiol Behav*, 93, 606-611.

[45] Iwata, J. LeDoux, J.E.; Meeley, M.P.; Arneric, S. & Reis, D.J. (1986). Intrinsic neurons in the amygdaloid field projected to by the medial geniculate body mediate emotional responses conditioned to acoustic stimuli. *Brain Res* , 383(1-2), 195 -214 .

[46] Jaber, M, Robinson, S. W, Missale, C, & Caron, M. G. (1996). Dopamine receptors and brain function. *Neuropharmacology*, 35, 1503-1519.

[47] Jacob, S, & Mcclintock, M. K. (2000). Psychological state and mood effects of steroidal chemosignals in women and men. *Horm Behav*, 37, 57-78.

[48] Karlson, P, & Lüscher, M. (1959). Pheromones: a new term for a class of biologically active substances. *Nature*, 183(4653), 55-56.

[49] Kessler, R. C, Ruscio, A. M, Shear, K, & Wittchen, H. U. (2010). Epidemiology of anxiety disorders. *Curr Top Behav Neurosci*, 2, 21-35.

[50] Kessler, M. S, Debilly, S, Schöppenthau, S, Bielser, T, Bruns, A, Künnecke, B, Kienlin, M, Wettstein, J. G, Moreau, J. L, & Risterucci, C. (2012). fMRI fingerprint of unconditioned fear-like behavior in rats exposed to trimethylthiazoline. *Eur Neuropsychopharmacol*, 22(3), 222-230.

[51] Kikusui, T, Takigami, S, Takeuchi, Y, & Mori, Y. (2001). Alarm pheromone enhances stress-induced hyperthermia in rats. *Physiol Behav*, 72(1-2), 45 .

[52] Kiyokawa, Y, Shimozuru, M, Kikusui, T, Takeuchi, Y, & Mori, Y. (2006). Alarm pheromone increases defensive and risk assessment behaviors in male rats. *Physiol Behav,* 87(2), 383-387.

[53] LaBar, K.S., & Cabeza, R. (2006). Cognitive neuroscience of emotional memory. *Nat Rev Neurosci,* 7(1), 54-64.

[54] Lang, P. J. (1995). The emotion probe: studies of motivation and attention. *Am Psychol,* 50, 372-385.

[55] Lázaro-Muñoz, G, LeDoux, J E, & Cain, C K. (2010). Sidman instrumental avoidance initially depends on lateral and basal amygdala and is constrained by central amygdala-mediated Pavlovian processes. *Biol Psychiatry,* 67, 1120-1127.

[56] LeDoux, J E. (2007). The amygdala. *Curr Biol,* 17, 868-874.

[57] LeDoux, J E. (2000). Emotion circuits in the brain. *Annu Rev Neurosci,* 23, 155-184.

[58] Lledo, P. M, Gheusi, G, & Vincent, J. D. (2005). Information processing in the mammalian olfactory system. *Physiol Rev,* 85, 281-317.

[59] Maren, S. (1999). Neurotoxic basolateral amygdala lesions impair learning and memory but not the performance of conditional fear in rats. *J Neurosci,* 19, 8696-8703.

[60] Maron, E, Nutt, D, & Shlik, J. (2012). Neuroimaging of serotonin system in anxiety disorders. *Curr Pharm Des,* in press.

[61] Martínez-Mota, L, Estrada-Camarena, E, López-Rubalcava, C, Contreras, C. M, & Fernández-Guasti, A. (2000). Interaction of desipramine with steroid hormones on experimental anxiety. *Psychoneuroendocrinology,* 25, 109-120.

[62] Mawson, A. R. (2005). Understanding mass panic and other collective responses to threat and disaster. *Psychiatry,* 68(2), 95-113.

[63] Maynard-Smith, J, & Harper, D. (2003). Animal signals. Oxford: Oxford University Press.

[64] Medina-Mora, M. E, Borges, G, Lara, C, Benjet, C, Blanco, J, Fleiz, C, Villatoro, J, Rojas, E, Zambrano, J, Casanova, L, & Aguilar-Gaxiola, S. (2003). Prevalencia de trastornos mentales y uso de servicios: resultados de la Encuesta Nacional de Epidemiología Psiquiátrica en México. *Salud Mental,* 26(4), 1-16.

[65] Menard, J, & Treit, D. (1999). Effects of centrally administered anxiolytic compounds in animal models of anxiety. *Neurosci Biobehav Rev,* 23(4), 591-613.

[66] Michelsson, K, Christensson, K, Rothgänger, H, & Winberg, J. (1996). Crying in separated and non-separated newborns: sound spectrographic analysis. *Acta Paediatrica,* 85(4), 471-475.

[67] Morilak, D. A, Barrera, G, Echevarria, D. J, García, A. S, Hernández, A, Ma, S, & Petre, C. O. (2005). Role of brain norepinephrine in the behavioral response to stress. *Prog Neuropsychopharmacol Biol Psychiatry,* 29(8), 1214-1224.

[68] Müller, M, & Fendt, M. (2006). Temporary inactivation of the medial and basolateral amygdala differentially affects TMT-induced fear behavior in rats. *Behav Brain Res*, 167, 57-62.

[69] Nader, K, Majidishad, P, Amorapanth, P, & LeDoux, J E. (2001). Damage to the lateral and central, but not other, amygdaloid nuclei prevents the acquisition of auditory fear conditioning. *Learn Mem*, 8, 156-163.

[70] Nemeroff, C. B. (2003a). Anxiolytics past, present, and future agents. *J Clin Psychiatry*, 64, 3 -6 .

[71] Nowak, R, Porter, R. H, Lévy, F, Orgeur, P, & Schaal, B. (2000). Role of mother-young interactions in the survival of offspring in domestic mammals. *Rev Reprod*, 5(3), 153-163.

[72] Nutt, D. J, & Malizia, A. L. (2001). New insights into the role of the $GABA_A$-benzodiazepine receptor in psychiatric disorders. *Br J Psychiatry*, 179(5), 390-396.

[73] Pani, L, Porcella, A, & Gessa, G. L. (2000). The role of stress in the pathophysiology of the dopaminergic system. *Mol Psychiatry*, 5(1), 14-21.

[74] Pastel, R. H. (2001). Collective behaviors: mass panic and outbreaks of multiple unexplained symptoms. *Mil Med*, 166(12), 44-46.

[75] Pauli, P, Marquardt, C, Hartl, L, Nutzinger, D. O, Hölzl, R, & Strian, F. (1991). Anxiety induced by cardiac perceptions in patients with panic attacks: a field study. *Behav Res Ther*, 29(2), 137-145.

[76] Pelletier, J. G, Likhtik, E, Filali, M, & Paré, D. (2005). Lasting increases in basolateral amygdala activity after emotional arousal: implications for facilitated consolidation of emotional memories. *Learn Mem*, 12, 96-102.

[77] Petrovich, G. D, Canteras, N. S, & Swanson, L. W. (2001). Combinatorial amygdalar inputs to hippocampal domains and hypothalamic behavior systems. *Brain Res Brain Res Rev*, 38(1-2), 247 -89 .

[78] Piñeyro, G, & Blier, P. (1999). Autoregulation of serotonin neurons: role in antidepressant drug action. *Pharmacol Rev*, 51(3), 533-591.

[79] Pinker, S, & Jackendoff, R. (2005). The faculty of language: what's special about it? *Cognition*, 95(2), 201-236.

[80] Porter, R. H, & Winberg, J. (1999). Unique salience of maternal breast odors for newborn infants. *Neurosci Biobehav Rev*, 23(3), 439-449.

[81] Regnier, F. E. (1971). Semiochemicals: structure and function. *Biol Reprod*, 4, 309-326.

[82] Romanski, L. M, & LeDoux, J E. (1992). Equipotentiality of thalamo-amygdala and thalamo-cortico-amygdala circuits in auditory fear conditioning. *J Neurosci*, 12(11), 4501-4509.

[83] Roozendaal, B, & Curt, P. (2000). Glucocorticoids and the regulation of memory consolidation. *Psychoneuroendocrinology*, 25, 213-238.

[84] Sah, P, Faber, E. S. L, Lopez de Armentia, M, & Power, J. (2003). The amygdaloid complex: anatomy and physiology. *Physiol Rev*, 83, 803-834.

[85] Schaal, B. (1988). Olfaction in infants and children: developmental and functional perspectives. *Chem Senses*, 13(2), 145-190.

[86] Serra, M, Pisu, M. G, Littera, M, Papi, G, Sanna, E, Tuveri, F, Usala, L, Purdy, R. H, & Biggio, G. (2000). Social isolation-induced decreases in both the abundance of neuroactive steroids and $GABA_A$ receptor function in rat brain. *J Neurochem*, 75(2), 732-740.

[87] Siever, L. J, Kahn, R. S, Lawlor, B. A, Trestman, R. L, Lawrence, T. L, & Coccaro, E. F. (1991). Critical issues in defining the role of serotonin in psychiatric disorders. *Pharmacol Rev*, 43(4), 509-525.

[88] Singh, O. P, Mandal, N, Biswas, A, Mondal, S, Sen, S, & Mukhopadhyay, S. (2009). An investigation into a mass psychogenic illness at Burdwan, West Bengal. *Indian J Public Health*, 53(1), 55-57.

[89] Sperling, W, Bleich, S, & Reulbach, U. (2008). Black Monday on stock markets throughout the world: a new phenomenon of collective panic disorder? A psychiatric approach. *Med Hypotheses*, 71(6), 972-974.

[90] Staples, L.G, Hunt, G.E, Cornish, J.L, & McGregor, I.S. (2005). Neural activation during cat odor-induced conditioned fear and "trial 2" fear in rats. *Neurosci Biobehav Rev*, 29(8), 1265-1277.

[91] Stout, S. C, Kilts, C. D, & Nemeroff, C. B. (1995). Neuropeptides and stress: preclinical findings and implication for pathophysiology. In: Friedman, M.J.; Charney, D.S. & Deutch, A.Y. (eds)., *Neurobiological and clinical consequences of stress: from normal adaptation to post-traumatic stress disorder*, 103-123, Philadelphia: Lippincott-Raven.

[92] Swanson, L. W, & Petrovich, G. D. (1998). What is the amygdala? *Trends Neurosci*, 21(8), 323-331.

[93] Takahashi, L. K, Hubbard, D. T, Lee, I, Dar, Y, & Sipes, S. M. (2007). Predator odor-induced conditioned fear involves the basolateral and medial amygdala. *Behav Neurosci*, 121, 100-110.

[94] Travis, M. J, & Bruce, T. (1994). Who cares for young carers? *BMJ*, 309(6950), 341.

[95] Tunçel, N, & Töre, F. C. (1998). The effect of vasoactive intestinal peptide (VIP) and inhibition of nitric oxide synthase on survival rate in rats exposed to endotoxin shock. *Ann N Y Acad Sci*, 865, 586-589.

[96] Uusi-oukari, M, & Korpi, E. R. (2010). Regulation of $GABA_A$ receptor subunit expression by pharmacological agents. *Pharmacol Rev*, 62(1), 97-135.

[97] Varendi, H, Christensson, K, Porter, R. H, & Winberg, J. (1998). Soothing effect of amniotic fluid smell in newborn infants. *Early Hum Development*, 51(1), 47-55.

[98] Varendi, H, Porter, R. H, & Winberg, J. (1996). Attractiveness of amniotic fluid odor: evidence of prenatal learning? *Acta Pediatrica*, 85(10), 1223-1227.

[99] Vermetthen, E, & Bremner, J. D. (2002). Circuits and systems in stress: I. Preclinical studies. *Depress Anxiety*, 15, 126-147.

[100] Vermetten, M. D, Charney, D. S, & Bremner, J. D. (2003). From anxiety disorders to PTSD. Vermetten, M.D. (ed)., *Posttraumatic stress disorder: neurobiological studies in the aftermath of traumatic stress*, 3-13, Utrecht: Remco Haringhuizen and Adriaan Kraal.

[101] Villarreal, G, & King, C. Y. (2001). Brain imaging in posttraumatic stress disorder. *Semin Clin Neuropsychiatry*, 6, 131-145.

[102] Xu, F, Schaefer, M, Kida, I, Schafer, J, Liu, N, Rothman, D. L, Hyder, F, Restrepo, D, & Shepherd, G. M. (2005). Simultaneous activation of mouse main and accessory olfactory bulbs by odors or pheromones. *J Comp Neurol*, 489, 491-500.

[103] Yamazaki, K, Beauchamp, G. K, Curran, M, Bard, J, & Boyse, E. A. (2000). Parent-progeny recognition as a function of MHC odor type identity. *Proc Natl Acad Sci U S A*, 97, 10500-10502.

[104] Zigmond, M. J, Castro, S. L, Keefe, K. A, Abercrombie, E. D, & Sved, A. F. (1998). Role of excitatory amino acids in the regulation of dopamine synthesis and release in the neostriatum. *Amino Acids*, 57 -62 .

Chapter 2

An Evolutionary Perspective on Anxiety and Anxiety Disorders

John Scott Price

Additional information is available at the end of the chapter

1. Introduction

Anxiety and depression are two of the negative emotions described by Levenson (1994). These emotions, along with anger, tend to disrupt the emotional homeostasis of the body, while the positive emotions such as contentment tend to restore homeostasis. The actions of anxiety and depression may be synergistic but they differ in important respects. Anxiety usually has an obvious cause and also a goal (safety, and the avoidance of danger), whereas depression usually has no obvious cause and also has no goal. Depression is thought to be related to social factors in relation to other human beings, whereas anxiety is related partly to social situations but also to non-social dangers. The strategies for dealing with human danger include submission, whereas this is not an appropriate response to non-human danger. Anxiety is classically thought to be concerned with the threat of danger, whereas depression is thought to be the result of danger. I will describe later how the negative emotions can be divided into the escalating emotions such as anger and the de-escalating emotions of anxiety and depression

In a recent monograph, Bruene (2008) says, "Behavioral observation of patients with anxiety disorders suggests that these disorders – as a group – reflect exaggerated responses to internal or external signals of perceived danger or threat. The autonomic part of the anxiety response pattern prepares the organism for one of several response options to terminate the anxiety-eliciting situation, namely, flight, immobility, submission or aggression."

An evolutionary approach to any behaviour (including anxiety and other forms of psychopathology) refers to two separate "causes". One is the question of function. What is the function of this behaviour, if any? Why has it evolved? What adaptive advantage does it give to the individual, or the individual's close kin, or to the individual's social group? This approach relies on behavioural ecology, which is the study of the function of behaviour, and the evolution of alternative behavioural strategies (Troisi, 2005). The other question is its phylogenetic origin. How did it evolve in our ancestors, and does it occur in other species? Clearly the fossil record does not record anxiety, and whether it occurs in our immediate-return hunter-gatherer ancestors has not been adequately studied. So the occurrence of anxiety in other species is of interest, bearing in mind that behaviour can be very different in closely related species, such as the absence or presence of paternal behaviour in some rodents (e.g., montane vs. prairie voles).

These two questions, the function of behaviour and its phylogenetic origin, are two of the four questions which Tinbergen famously asked of any behaviour in order to understand it properly (Tinbergen, 1963): What is its function, what is its phylogeny, what is its ontogeny, what is its immediate causation? Of course, statements about the function of a behaviour during evolution are in a different logical category from statements about proximal causation, in that they cannot be verified empirically. This has led to negative comments from some sources (e.g. Dubrovsky, 2002), caricaturing them as "just-so stories", in the same category as Rudyard Kipling's "How the leopard got its spots"; but if we did not ask how the leopard got its spots, we might know a lot less about camouflage, colour vision and predator-prey relations,

I wrote on this topic ten years ago, and since what I said than can be read free on the internet (Price, 2003) I will try not to repeat myself, but rather emphasise certain points and attempt to cover more recent thinking.

2. The adaptive function of anxiety

It is obvious that anxiety is adaptive in protecting the individual from danger. A person who crossed Niagara Falls on a tightrope every day would not last long. In the UK we have had many deaths from "tombstoning", which means jumping off a high cliff into water (and entering it vertically, like a tombstone). Anxious avoidance of snakes and spiders has clearly saved lives, and the fact that there is no in-built anxiety about cars and electric sockets indicates that evolution has not had time to build up anxiety about these dangers. This is because of a "mismatch" between the present and the Era of Evolutionary Adaptation (EEA), which is the evolutionary time in which adaptations evolved.

I will write about the triune brain (McLean, 1990; Ploog, 2003). Although Paul McLean's ideas have been trashed by his successors in neuroanatomy (Wikipedia), and they do not fit well with the neuroanatomy of vocalisation (Newman, 2002), I think that some of his ideas are helpful, especially his idea of the forebrain consisting of three "central processing assemblies", operating somewhat independently, and arranged in a rostro-caudal sequence in the mammalian forebrain. This triune brain may well underlie the triune mind postulated by philosophers such as Plato, Pascal and Gurdjieff. Although I discussed this matter ten years ago, there is more to be said. One important finding is that the genetic tendency to generalised anxiety disorder (GAD) and major depressive disorder is the same (Kendler et al., 1992; Hettema et al., 2005), and so from an evolutionary view the arguments for one apply also to the other. My own view is that anxiety and depression operate synergistically to manage social change in small groups, but more of that in a later section.

First, I will illustrate how escalation and de-escalation can be hypothesised to occur relatively independently at the three levels of the triune brain. Each level makes its own decision, when confronted by a threat or challenge, either to escalate or de-escalate:

Brain level	Response	to	threat
	Escalate	or	De-escalate
Rational level (isocortex)	Decide to fight (stubbornness or courage)	or	Decide to flee or submit (common sense)
Emotional level (limbic system)	Anger, feel assertive and confident	or	ANXIETY, feel inferior , impotent,
Instinctive level (basal ganglia)	Elevated mood	or	Depressed mood Anxious mood, GAD

Table 1. Escalating and de-escalating strategies at three brain levels: agonistic competition.

Human competition is very different from animal competition, and most of the methods of competition do not involve face-to-face encounters with rivals. Moreover, success is achieved not by intimidating a rival, but by attracting positive responses from other members of the group, resulting in prestige. Remarkably, the choices between escalation and de-escalation have survived the transition from agonistic to prestige competition, and so we can emend Table 1 to express the new type of competition, as laid out in Table 2:

Brain level	Response	to	competition
	Escalate	or	De-escalate
Rational level (isocortex)	Adopt new goals, actively pursue existing goals, assert oneself, speak in public	or	Give up goals, efface oneself, refrain from public speaking
Emotional level (limbic system)	Feel assertive, exhilarated and enthusiastic	or	ANXIETY, feel inferior, ashamed, writer's block
Instinctive level (basal ganglia)	Elevated mood	or	Depressed mood Anxious mood, GAD

Table 2. Escalating and de-escalating strategies at three brain levels: prestige competition.

It should be clear that de-escalation at the rational level can pre-empt or terminate de-escalation at the lower levels. These lower levels have evolved as a safety net in case the rational brain is too ambitious. Therefore we often see patients who are escalating at the rational level, but, their escalation being unsuccessful, the lower levels are accessed. We also see patients who are escalating at the emotional level, and in spite of de-escalation at the rational level, if the angry emotion does not achieve its aim, we then get de-escalation at the instinctive level. Most of these patients have suffered unjustified misfortune, such as death of a child or being passed over in work by an incompetent member of the family firm; they are denied the principle of retributive justice, as was Job in the Book of Job of the Old Testament.

The idea of separating the negative emotions into escalatory and de-escalatory is not new. Stone (2002) reports that "Maurice de Fleury (1897) divided the emotions into two groups. Doubt, humility, sloth, fearfulness, sadness and pity are symptoms – to varying degrees – of cerebral exhaustion; Pride, foolishness, anger, egoism, courage, heroism, and cruelty are the manifestations of exaltation of the spirit." (p. 9).

2.1. The anxiety-generating effect of bad news

I would like to re-emphasise the importance of "bad news" in the genesis of psychopathology, as this does not seem to be generally recognised. Bad news, of deaths and other disasters, is not available to our primate cousins who are not equipped to exchange gossip, but has been available to our ancestors over the last few million years since language evolved. Since these ancestors lived in groups of about 150 individuals, the amount of bad news they could generate was limited, even if we add in bad news from neighbouring groups. Now, we have available the bad news of many billions of people. Since news of death or other disaster may presage the nearby existence of a predator or of raiding parties from neighbouring tribes, or of disease, it must have been adaptive for bad news to increase anxiety and promote activities to ward off occurrence, such as increased washing, checking of security arrangements, and the advantageous territorial constriction of agoraphobia.

In the EEA bad news was probably discussed and so shared with other group members, whereas modern man tends to watch it or listen to it on his own, or at least without comment. Things are worse when the bad news is close by. An Egyptian psychiatrist (Nagy, 2012) reports on a patient who was glued to her TV set, absorbing the chaos all around her; and the situation was dire: two of the psychiatrist's students were killed while trying to save injured protesters.

When I practiced as a clinician, I advised all my anxious patients to avoid watching TV news, and I found that many of them had learned the lesson for themselves. They realised that each item of bad news raised their background level of anxiety, and, of course, severely depressed patients may believe that they are personally responsible for the disasters which occur daily around the globe.

There is a need for controlled study of the effect of reducing patients' access to bad news, and this is difficult in modern conditions when family television has replaced games and conversation for family interaction. I make a point of advising my anxious patients to restrict their viewing to comedies and nature programmes, although this injunction may cause family arguments, if other members of the family have a different viewing agenda. This is yet another argument for treating patients in family groups, so that the whole family can be motivated to protect the patient from the horrors of contemporary life. No one, to my knowledge, has done a controlled trial of "news avoidance" as an item of therapy.

2.2. Growing up with anxiety

A lot of variation in neuroticism (the personality equivalent of anxiety-proneness) is due to genetic factors and to non-shared environmental experience, negating the folk psychology view that children are strongly influenced by the behaviour of their parents and the atmosphere of the family home. Some genotypes prosper under negative home circumstances, whereas others suffer under those circumstances, but prosper more than the "tough ones" when the environment is benign (Bruene et al., 2012). This confirms the old observation that some children do better with the stick, and others with the carrot. We need to improve our means of distinguishing these two genotypes early in childhood.

I will say something about the genesis of anxiety in adolescence. Much good work has been done on the establishment of a secure base for the child in infancy (Price, 2000), but less has been done on adolescence, which in my clinical experience is a strong divider into the happy and the miserable. Some young people take to adolescence like a duck to water, and they are accepted by their adolescent peers and given positions of influence and even leadership in their groups. Others do badly at this time, and are bullied unmercifully by both boys and girls, that by boys tending to be physical, that by girls tending towards social exclusion. Normal children entering adolescence may be disadvantaged for many reasons; they may be odd in some way, speak with an unusual accent, have some physical deformity, or maybe they have moved into an area where the adolescent group is already full and does not want new recruits. For those who have suffered anxious or avoidant attachment in infancy, the problems of adolescence are compounded (Wilson, Price & Preti, 2009).

2.3. Social anxiety disorder (SAD)

Social anxiety disorder (SAD) is an exaggeration of the normal submissive or appeasement display which people make to more powerful individuals or to a disapproving group. Kaminer and Stein (2005) point out that SAD is an excessive fear of humiliating or embarrassing oneself while being exposed to public scrutiny or to unfamiliar people, resulting in intense anxiety upon exposure to social performance situations. Feared social situations are either avoided as much as possible or create significant distress. Physical manifestations of anxiety in the feared situations include a shaky voice, clammy hands, tremors and blushing. In the generalized sub-type of SAD, anxiety is associated with most social situations (including both formal performance situations such as giving a speech or speaking at a meeting, and informal social interactions such as initiating conversations, attending parties or dating); in the non-generalized sub-type, anxiety occurs only in specific social situations, such as public speaking, or eating/drinking in public, or writing in public. Prevalence rates for SAD range from 3% to 16%. From an evolutionary point of view, SAD must promote group functioning by reducing social competition, and ensuring that group discussions in the council chamber do not last indefinitely. Most readers will be aware that in question time after a scientific paper, the people who ask questions are those who have social confidence and like the sound of their own voices, regardless of their knowledge of the subject, whereas many of those with something important to say remain silent because of SAD.

3. Anxiety in other species

Anxiety is the emotion associated with avoidance of danger, and it is obvious that many species encounter more danger than ourselves. Humans are sometimes taken by tigers and other predators, but many species are subject to constant predation, being the basic diet of the predator species. Can we learn from their reactions? One obvious defensive measure is to have a safe haven, especially at night. Some species avoid danger by being enclosed, others by being exposed. An extreme example of being enclosed is the naked mole rat, which does not appear above the surface of the earth. Rabbits avoid danger to their young by visiting them for suckling only once a day, and ferrets are more extreme in suckling only once in 48 hours. In this way they avoid giving predators a clue as to the whereabouts of their burrow, and this advantage clearly outweighs the advantage of constant maternal care. When kept in cages, rabbit and ferret mothers cannot do this, which may account for some of the aggressiveness they show at this time. Some species prefer to be exposed, such as the hamadryas baboon which sleeps on a cliff face, and many birds nest on cliffs for the same reason. Some humans adopt both strategies, and live in caves which open onto the cliff face, and in this case either acrophobia or claustrophobia would be a disadvantage.

A lot of information about animal anxiety is available informally on the internet: just Google "anxiety in horses (or monkeys, or birds, etc.)". Different animals have different sources of anxiety and different reactions to it; for instance, horses suffer from severe separation anxiety, and this no doubt originated in their need to stay with their herd.

Some group-living species delegate the role of anxious individual to one of their members, so that the rest can forage free from anxiety. We have all seen films of meerkats in which the group forages happily while one member stands on a mound and looks anxiously for birds of prey and terrestrial predators. This delegation of responsibility may be important for humans. If a foraging meerkat does not trust the sentry, the freedom from anxiety may be lost. If the obsessional housewife does not trust her cleaning lady, she is likely to repeat the work while nursing pathological grievance against her employee.

3.1. Phylogeny of anxiety

In an intriguing chapter, Hofer (2002) describes the response to danger in organisms of varying complexity. The bacterium swims forward with its flagella working together, absorbing molecules of sucrose and other foodstuffs. However, if receptors on its surface detect a toxin, its flagella then act independently, and the bacterium tumbles about. In half a second, it has forgotten about the toxin and sets off with flagella all pulling together, in whatever direction it happens to be pointing at the time. Hofer comments: "When it stops and tumbles in response to the presence of a negative signal, is it anxious? Certainly, we would not want to say so, even though the mental picture of a tumbling creature with flagellar hairs standing on end may be intuitively persuasive.....The presence of these behaviors in so primitive an organism gives us an idea of how basic a state resembling anxiety has been for survival of life forms."

Hofer also discusses the invertebrate sea hare, *Aplysia californicus*. It can be conditioned to respond with avoidance to shrimp juice by associating it with electric shocks (mimicking its predator, the starfish), thus producing a state of anticipatory anxiety, but in the absence of shrimp juice (the conditioned stimulus) its behaviour is normal. However, a series of uncontrollable electric shocks produces a "persistent state (lasting several weeks) in which defensive and escape responses were exaggerated, and responses to positive events were blunted, an abnormal behavioral repertoire had been established that resembled a form of chronic diffuse anxiety."

The development of the limbic system in mammals allowed new and social forms of anxiety to evolve. Rat pups emit high frequency squeaks when separated from their mother and these sounds release searching and retrieval behaviour in the mother. In his own work, Hofer was able to breed strains of rats with high and low tendency to emit squeaks. He speculates that the ability to squeak evolved to keep the rats warm, and only secondarily became a signal to the mother (exaptation). The squeaks are inhibited by benzodiazepines and opioids, and exacerbated by benzodiazepine antagonists. In later work (Brunelli & Hofer, 2007) the high squeak infant rats developed into nervous adults, while the low squeak rats were notable for their aggression, so there had presumably been selection for escalation versus de-escalation in the emotional (limbic) forebrain. Presumably, rabbit and ferret pups do not respond to separation in this way, otherwise they would attract predators to their burrow.

Turning to primates, Hofer describes Suomi's work on free-ranging rhesus macaques on an island in the Caribbean. This population contained a sub-population of very anxious individuals, some of whom suffered from "lasting incapacitating states resulting in substantial mortality". The anxious traits could be increased by selective breeding and prevention of good mothering. He describes the response to "chronically threatening conditions. Persistent anxiety (high levels of arousal, searching for cues for danger, and high levels of avoidance of potentially damaging encounters) confers an adaptive advantage over less anxious individuals." There has been criticism of Suomi's work on humanitarian grounds.

In the case of humans, Hofer describes the speculation of Klein that panic attacks may be a response to imminent suffocation, mediated by high levels of blood carbon dioxide. Hyperventilation (overbreathing) is a common feature of panic attacks, and may aggravate the panic by causing tetany due to low levels of carbon dioxide and thus an excessively alkaline blood.

My own extensive experience of patients with panic attacks resulted from an appointment as medical casualty officer in a hospital near an underground railway station in London. Two or three patients a day were brought by ambulance from the station, having developed panic in the underground, especially when it was crowded and the train stopped between stations. These patients had very rapid respirations which caused involuntary contraction of muscles and sensations of tingling due to the alkalinity of the blood due to loss of carbonic acid due to overbreathing. Of course, these symptoms aggravated the panic and most of the patients thought they were dying. Their condition was rapidly cured by getting them to breathe into a paper bag, so that they were rebreathing their own carbon dioxide. Talking to these patients when they had recovered, it was clear that most of them were healthy young adults who had no history of excessive anxiety or any other psychiatric disorder.

Hofer concludes by pointing out that patients may benefit by being told that they are suffering from, not madness, but from a mechanism that has enabled their ancestors to survive the dangers of our evolutionary past.

4. Genetics

A lot of excitement has been caused by the discovery of a polymorphism in the serotonin transporter gene (which enables the reuptake of serotonin into the presynaptic neuron),because most of our effective antidepressant drugs inhibit the reuptake of serotonin. Equally exciting is the possibility that there is a gene/environment interaction in its effect (Risch et al., 2009). It has been suggested that the "short" allele of the serotonin transporter coding gene is associated with greater risk for depression if linked with early childhood adversities, yet the same version of the gene is associated with *reduced* risk for depression if carriers grow up in emotionally secure conditions (Belsky & Pluess, 2009). This suggests that selection favoured plasticity or "open programs" that render individuals more susceptible to environmental contingencies – for better *and* worse (Belsky, Jonassaint & Pluess, 2009). Similarly, psychiatrists guided by evolutionary theory have recognized that antagonistic pleiotropy may play a role in psychiatric disorders – genes that convey fitness advantages in one domain, while having potentially maladaptive value in another domain, a concept that was originally put forth with regard to senescence (Bruene et al., 2012). Nowadays, examples for antagonistic pleiotropy can be pinned down to even single genes such as the catecholamine-O-methyltransferase coding gene, of which one particular allele is associated with poorer working memory performance but superior empathy (Heinz & Smolka, 2006)). Taken together, these insights offer an answer to the question of why natural selection designed bodies that are – under specific circumstances – vulnerable to disease (Nesse & Williams, 1994). There have been several hundred studies of the serotonin transporter gene in various psychiatric populations and consistent results are not easy to obtain (Duncan & Keller, 2010).

I mentioned above some findings from the large Virginia twin study carried out by Kendler and his colleagues (Hettema, Prescott, Myers et al., 2005). They found that the genetic predisposition to major depressive disorder was the same as that to generalised anxiety disorder and to panic disorder. There was some overlap with social anxiety disorder and agoraphobia, but the genetic predisposition to specific phobias was separate. This means that if one is predisposed by genetics to major depressive disorder, one is equally predisposed to general anxiety disorder (GAD), but the same cannot be said for lesser degrees of anxiety.

4.1. The serotonin transporter gene in macaques.

Humans and macaques are the only primates to have the short version of the serotonin transporter gene. 48% of Caucasian populations are heterozygotes, having both short and long alleles. 36% are homozygotes for the long allele, 16% for the short allele. Rhesus monkeys who possess the short allele are notably more anxious than the long homozygotes (Watson et al., 2009). Moreover, when shown pictures of dominant monkeys, their pupils dilate more than those who are homozygous for the long allele, and they have to be bribed (with juice) to see the face of a dominant monkey, whereas the long homozygotes will forego juice in order to see the same pictures. The rearing of these monkeys is not described, so it is difficult to compare with the human data mentioned above.

4.2. Anxiety in different human cultures

I am not an anthropologist, but it is clear from the literature that some cultures have different attitudes to anxiety and maybe different genetic predispositions. Margaret Mead (1935) studied three tribes living in the Sepik River Valley of Papua New Guinea. The Mundugumor were very aggressive and warlike, so that anxiety was not a desirable feature with them (but the actual frequency of anxiety is not known). The Arapesh were extremely peaceful. The Tchambuli were also peaceful and the men spent their time putting on plays. The two latter tribes had been driven out of the fertile areas of the island.

The Tarahumara of Mexico (McDougall, 2010) are reported to be extremely nervous and inhibited, so that any social contact requires large quantities of corn beer to be consumed. They are famous for their utrarunning (running more than marathon distances), and possibly they seek the "runner's high" (thought to be due to the release of endogenous opioids) to counter their natural timidity.

Also very nervous are the Chewong of the Malaysian Peninsular, and in this tribe the admired norm of behaviour is to be timid (Howell, 2012). It is said that the elders are fond of telling stories about the times they have run away. Asiatics may have higher frequencies of the short version of the serotonin transporter gene than Europeans (Watson et al., 2009).

5. Anxiety and its resolution in a sacred text

For reasons of confidentiality, we cannot present case histories from our practice, but fortunately there is a clear account of an anxiety attack and its resolution in the Hindu epic poem, the Mahabharata (Price& Gardner, 2009). The poem describes a long and bitter struggle between two sets of cousins, the Pandavas and Kauravas, for control of ancestral lands. The Bhagavad Gita (a small part of the Mahabharata) begins with the two armies drawn up for battle with warriors blowing conches and beating drums. Arjuna, a younger Pandava brother renowned as an archer, drives his chariot between the armies to assess the opposition. His charioteer is none other than the god Sri Krishna. As Arjuna views the superior Kaurava army, he sees relatives and mentors he knows well. He feels doubts about killing these family members and friends, translated by Mitchell (2002) as follows:

Arjuna saw them standing there: fathers, grandfathers, teachers, uncles, brothers, sons, grandsons, fathers-in-law, and friends, kinsmen on both sides, each arrayed against the other. In despair, overwhelmed with pity, he said: "As I see my own kinsmen, gathered here, eager to fight, my legs weaken, my mouth dries, my body trembles, my hair stands on end, my skin burns, the bow Gandiva drops from my hand. I am beside myself, my mind reels. I see evil omens, Krishna; no good can come from killing my own kinsmen in battle. I have no desire for victory or for the pleasures of kingship" ..... Having spoken these words, Arjuna sank down into the chariot and dropped his arrows and bow, his mind heavy with grief.....

As Arjuna sat there, overwhelmed with pity, desperate, tears streaming from his eyes, Krishna spoke these words to him: "Why this timidity, Arjuna, at a time of crisis? It is unworthy of a noble mind; it is shameful and does not lead to heaven. This cowardice is beneath you, Arjuna; do not give in to it. Shake off your weakness. Stand up now like a man."

Arjuna said: "When the battle begins, how can I shoot arrows through Bhishma and Drona, who deserve my reverence? ...... I am weighted down with pity, Krishna; my mind is utterly confused. Tell me where my duty lies, which path I should take. I am your pupil; I beg you for your instruction. For I cannot imagine how any victory – even if I were to gain the kingship of the whole earth or of all the gods in heaven – could drive away this grief that is withering my senses."

Having spoken thus to Krishna, Arjuna said: "I will not fight," and fell silent.

As Arjuna sat there, downcast, between the two armies, Krishna smiled at him, then spoke ...

The god Krishna, the eighth avatar of Vishnu, then speaks to Arjuna for 16 more chapters (and the reader is left to wonder what the two armies are doing during this time). In a verbal dominance display of unparalleled beauty (except possibly for the speech of the Lord out of the whirlwind in the book of Job), Krishna explains to Arjuna that he is all-powerful, and then he displays himself to Arjuna in all his divine majesty. Arjuna is overwhelmed and submits to Krishna, saying "I will do as you command". He then recovers from his anxiety attack and fights heroically in the ensuing battle.

In this example we see a distressing situation lead to a severe panic attack, a request for advice which is not followed, a dominance display by the god followed by total submission on the part of Arjuna and then recovery from anxiety. By abrogating responsibility to Krishna at the rational level of his triune mind, Arjuna no longer needs the anxiety which arose from his emotional mind due to the initial failure of the rational mind to deal with the problem (by taking Krishna's advice).

5.1. Anxiety and art

Although artists can portray frightening scenes, it is less easy for them to depict the anxiety response. Here is a comment by Edvard Munch about his famous (and expensive) painting "The Scream":

"I was walking down the road with two friends when the sun set; suddenly, the sky turned as red as blood. I stopped and leaned against the fence, feeling unspeakably tired. Tongues of fire and blood stretched over the bluish black fjord. My friends went on walking, while I lagged behind, shivering with fear. Then I heard the enormous, infinite scream of nature." He later described the personal anguish behind the painting, "for several years I was almost mad... You know my picture, 'The Scream?' I was stretched to the limit—nature was screaming in my blood... After that I gave up hope ever of being able to love again." (Wikipedia).

5.2. Social presentation of the anxious person

Anxious patients may not appear anxious to others, but may be seen as aloof or even arrogant. Leahy (2010) puts it as follows::

"People with social phobia or social anxiety often give out signals of their own apprehension that inadvertently send the wrong message. For example, many of my patients over the years with social anxiety often don't smile, they avoid eye contact, and they remain silent because they are so anxious that they will either sound foolish or look anxious. Ironically, these attempts to remain "closed" result in the "wrong impression". Many of these people appear to be cold and aloof-and, in some cases, conceited. It's the wrong message and they don't even know they are sending it. Ironically, they fear that they will appear anxious, but they actually appear arrogant. They also fail to "mirror" or "match" the emotions that others are displaying. For example, other people may be smiling, but the anxious person may remain cool and aloof. This sends the wrong message - that you are not interested and you don't care."

One of my first patients was just such a young man, seen as aloof by fellow patients in a neurosis unit (Sainsbury and Price, 1969). Asked to paint "Myself and the group" in art therapy, he drew a circle of red blobs representing the group and a single black blob representing himself. In the group discussion the next day, the other patients said that they had thought he felt himself superior to them, but in the ensuing discussion he disabused them of this idea and was then accepted by the group. This is similar to the misperception of depressed patients, who are seen, not as depressed, but as lazy because they do not perform tasks well, or rude because they do not carry out social obligations such as writing thank-you letters.

The concealment of anxiety is a promising line of study. A chimpanzee in a conflict situation has been seen literally wiping the submissive grin off his face with his hand. Some tribes cut the muscles around the mouth to prevent the manifestation of a trembling lip. The concealment and detection of anxiety is to be found expressed in the novels of Georgette Hayer. Anxious young people may hide their anxiety from their parents, perhaps hiding scars on their forearms with long sleeves, and this may lead to further parental pressure to succeed academically which, of course, makes the anxiety worse. I described this situation in some detail in my previous paper (Price, 2003), and here I reproduce the figure which illustrates how the ambitious parents mistake the position of their child on the Yerkes-Dodson curve:

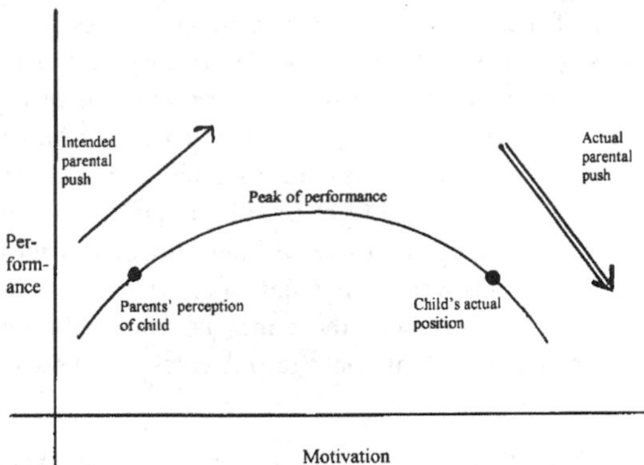

Figure 1. The inverted U-shaped curve of the Yerkes-Dosdon law. The single-shafted arrow represents the parents' attempt to push the child up towards the peak of performance. The double-shafted arrow represents the actual effect of the parental pushing.

6. Conclusion

Since evolutionary speculations are not directly testable, I have tried to show how they may be useful in planning treatment programmes, and in research. One of the main contributions of the evolutionary perspective is to show that anxiety plays a major role not only in protecting people from non-social dangers, but also in maintaining social stability in social groups. Practically all group-living vertebrates have social hierarchies which function to maintain peaceful relations within groups and also to provide a structure for social selection to occur. There is an enormous amount of inhibition in these animal groups, and this is maintained by anxiety and depression. Especially among males, life is one of continual inhibition, in which desires for mating, food and sleeping quarters are supressed. Few individuals achieve the alpha position in their groups, and it is only these alphas who are free to express their personalities and desires without inhibition. The acceptance of relatively low hierarchical position by other group members allows the group to work co-operatively, as in hunting by wolves and cape hunting dogs.

6.1. Rational de-escalation can prevent or terminate sub-rational de-escalation

Aristotle pointed out that if someone hits you, you experience pain; if the pain is caused by a higher ranking individual, you feel sad, if it is caused by a lower-ranking individual, you feel angry. You have no choice about these reactions as they are determined by the sub-rational brain. You do have a choice about your voluntary action. You can attack the person who hit you, and this is the fight version of the fight/flight response; or you can shrink away, and this is the flight version of the fight/flight response. If you attack a higher-ranking person, you are likely to incur severe costs; on the other hand, if you win, you stand to gain significant benefit. Since fight involves actions such as recruitment of allies, preparation of armaments and planning of strategy, it has been described as an escalatory response by behavioural ecologists; this contrasts with the de-escalatory response of flight which also includes submission, in which there may be not only an absence of flight, but an actual approach to the rival for the purpose of reconciliation. Therefore in a threat situation we have a choice between escalating and de-escalating strategies at two or more levels. With our rational brain we can choose either to fight or submit, and with our sub-rational brain we can "choose" either to feel angry or to feel sad and anxious. If these two brain levels choose the same strategy, then all is well, there is either angry attack or anxious submission. But if the two levels make opposite choices, there may be trouble. Especially if the rational brain decides on escalation and the subrational brain decides on de-escalation, we are in for trouble (psychopathology).

We do not have to go further than Charles Darwin himself for an example. His theory of evolution by natural selection was an attack not only on the church, but also on his wife (who held religious views). In pursuing his theory he was escalating at the rational level. His escalation was at first muted, since he kept his manuscript in a drawer for many years. But his attachment to the goal of publication was evidenced by his rapid response when a rival appeared in the form of Wallace, and he was quick to summarise his theory for joint presentation with Wallace to the Linnean Society. With encouragement from his friends, his rational response was escalation. But his sub-rational brain made a different analysis of the situation, seeing the church as a formidable rival and not one to be trifled with; therefore it made a decision to de-escalate. As a result Darwin was plagued with anxiety and psychosomatic symptoms for the rest of his life.

I have treated many patients who are escalating at the rational level but de-escalating at the sub-rational level. Reasons for rational escalation can be called courage or stubbornness, depending on your viewpoint. Moral scruples are a common cause for escalation; for instance, patients refuse to take part in stealing by fellow employees and so suffer social exclusion; one patient of mine refused to accept advertisements for call girls for her magazine, which put her in conflict with management. In our monograph, Stevens and I report in some detail the case of a porter who refused to take sick leave when he was not sick. The poet Milton (not a patient of mine!) continued writing poetry and tracts criticising the monarchy, and suffered ill-health as a consequence.

As can be seen from the Tables, the sub-rational brain can be divided into two, an emotional level in which there is partial realisation of the situation and an instinctive level in which there is no such realisation. Here again, escalation in the form of anger may be combined with de-escalation at a lower level in the form of depression and anxiety. If anger is effective in righting the situation, all is well, but often anger is frustrated by authority or by the situation itself, so that lower level de-escalation becomes chronic. Patients of mine in this situation include parents whose child had been killed by a drunken driver, people unjustly sacked form their jobs, parents whose children have been denied educational opportunity be the school system, and, in one remarkable case, a father whose daughter had precocious puberty and who was accused by social services of sexually interfering with her. Treatment in these cases is difficult. In some cases I have helped the patient to discharge the anger by writing letters to the offending authority. In some cases, joining a group with other people similarly abused can direct the anger into productive channels, as when group of parents whose children have been killed by drunken drivers band together to tighten the laws on drunken driving.

6.2. Delegation and abrogation

One clear suggestion from the evolutionary viewpoint is the desirability of shedding responsibility. This can take the form of delegation of responsibility to other members of the social group, and the model here is the adoption of the role of sentry by foraging meerkats. Also there is abrogation of responsibility to a more powerful person or a higher power. This is part of the programme of AA in which one "step" is to acknowledge that one cannot give up alcohol on one's own, without the help of a higher power, which may be some form of deity or an emergent property of the group. We have seen how Arjuna's panic attack and anxiety about killing his relatives and friends was allayed by submission to his God, Krishna. Many religions offer peace and joy to those who submit. One of my own anxieties is about the loss of rainforest in the world, and this anxiety is assuaged by my knowledge that Prince Charles is not only more worried about it than I am, but is also immensely more powerful.

The mismatch between the environment in which we evolved (the EEA) and the conditions we now live in are not difficult to apprehend. One crucial difference is the transmission of bad news. We now have daily reports of the tragedies and afflictions which affect many billions of people, whereas our ancestors knew only about the reverses suffered by a group of 150 or so people. Therefore it is sensible to encourage anxious people to avoid reading newspapers and watching news broadcasts, and stick to sport, comedy or nature programmes.

An evolutionary approach is also helpful for research, offering a wide variety of animal models of anxiety for the investigation of mechanisms and the testing of anxiolytics. There has been too little work on reptiles, some of whom change colour when defeated. Tail-chasing in dogs is being used as an animal model of obsessive-compulsive disorder (Tira et al., 2012).

6.3. Treating the anxious patient

Here is a check-list for the therapist who is treating an anxious patient:

1. Since from an evolutionary perspective anxiety is an unconscious form of submission, has the patient submitted consciously and voluntarily where necessary?

2. If the patient is a believer, have they submitted totally to their god, or are there elements of "My will be done", or is there a problem with accepting a god who allows unnecessary suffering? If the patient is not a believer, has he accepted the universe and his place in it: if not, he should join a group of people with similar problems.
3. At work, does she respect her boss, or does she think she could do the job better? Does she have insubordinate subordinates?
4. Has he or she submitted to the reasonable demands of the marriage partner?
5. Has he submitted to the rules of society? E.g., does he avoid paying taxes or fiddle his expenses?
6. Has the patient delegated where possible, and does he or she trust the person delegated to?
7. Has the patient restricted television viewing to comedy and nature programmes?
8. Have you spoken to the patient's marriage partner or someone else close to the patient? Teenage or grown up children often see things that adults miss, and they usually appreciate being involved in their parent's treatment, especially if there have been threats of suicide.
9. Is the anxiety worse after receiving letters or phone calls or visits from anyone?
10. Has the patient got supportive friends? If not, group therapy should be considered (and also for patients who have been abused by the adolescent peer group – fellow group members can provide a re-run of the adolescent experience).
11. Are the patient's goals in life realistic?
12. Is there conflict with anyone such as a neighbour or relative?
13. Is there unresolved grief?
14. Is there a problem with alcohol or anxiolytic medication?

In the behavioural treatment of anxiety, there is an odd situation in which extremes may be more beneficial than anything in between. Thus the choice may be between very gentle deconditioning and flooding, in which the patient is kept in the anxiety-arousing situation for as long as it takes for the anxiety to subside, and then the patient realises they can be in that situation without anxiety. This is similar to the situation with autistic children, with whom success has been achieved either by a very gradual approach or by overwhelming cuddling. The same applies to self-esteem, which may be built up with the help of a therapist, or the self may be abnegated to facilitate total submission to God. Philosophers advise us to take the middle course, but sometimes the middle course is ineffective.

In summary, anxiety evolved to keep us out of danger, to obey the rules of our group, and to treat each other with respect. If we have too much anxiety, we suffer, if we have too little, we may become insufferable.

Author details

John Scott Price

Retired psychiatrist, UK

References

[1] Belsky, J., & Pluess, M. (2009). Beyond diathesis stress: differential susceptibility to environmental influences. Psychological Bulletin, , 135, 885-908.

[2] Belsky, J., Jonassaint, C., Pluess, M., et al. (2009). Vulnerability genes or plasticity genes? Molecular Psychiatry , 14, 746-754.

[3] Brunelli, S., & Hofer, M. (2007). Selective breeding for infant rat separation-induced ultrasonic vocalizations: Developmental precursors of passive and active coping styles. *Behavioural Brain Research,* 182(2), 193-207.

[4] DOI: 10.1016/j.bbr.2007.04.014

[5] Brüne, M. (2008). Textbook of evolutionary psychiatry. The origins of psychopathology. Oxford: Oxford University Press.

[6] Brüne, M., Belsky, J., Fabrega, H., Feierman, J. R., Gilbert, P., Glantz, K., Polimeni, J., Price, J. S., Sanjuan, J., Sullivan, R., Troisi, A., & Wilson, D. R. (2012). The crisis of psychiatry- insights and prospects from evolutionary theory. World Psychiatry, 11 (1), 55-58.

[7] Dubrovsky, B. (2002). Evolutionary psychiatry: adaptationist and nonadaptationist conceptualisations. Progress in Neuro-Psychopharmacology & Biological Psychiatry, , 26, 1-19.

[8] Duncan, L. E., & Keller, M. C. (2011). A Critical Review of the First 10 Years of Candidate Gene-by-Environment Interaction Research in Psychiatry. American Journal of Psychiatrydoi:10.1176/appi.ajp.2011.11020191.PMC 3222234. PMID 21890791. // www.pubmedcentral.nih.gov/articlerender.fcgi?tool=pmcentrez&artid=3222234., 168, 1041-1049.

[9] Heinz, A., & Smolka, M. N. (2006). The effects of catechol-O-methyltransferase genotype on brain activation elicited by affective stimuli and cognitive tasks. Revue of Neuroscience, , 17, 359-367.

[10] Hettema JM, Prescott CA, Myers JM, Neale MC, Kendler KS. (2005). The structure of genetic and environmental risk factors for anxiety disorders in men and women. *Archives of General Psychiatry,* 182-189.

[11] Hofer, M. A. (2002). Evolutionary concepts of anxiety, In: Textbook of Anxiety Disorders, D.J.Stein & E.Hollander, (Eds.), American Psychiatric Publishing Inc., Washington, DC., 57-69.

[12] Howell, S. L. (2012). Cumulative Understandings: Experiences from the Study of Two Southeast Asian Societies, In Aud Talle & Signe Lise Howell (ed.), Returns to the Field. Indiana University Press. 978-0-25322-348-7Del 2, Chapter 6. s , 153-180.

[13] Kaminer, D., & Stein, D. J. (2005). An evolutionary perspective on SAD. CNSforum 14 Feb 2005http://kortlink.dk/cnsforum_SAD/map

[14] Kendler, K. S., Neale, M. C., Kessler, R. C., Heath, A. C., & Eaves, L. J. (1992). Major depression and generalized anxiety disorder. Same genes, (partly) different environments? *Archives of General Psychiatry*, 49, 716-722.

[15] Leahy, R.L(2010). Simple and powerful techniques for coping with anxiety and worry. Psychology Today, Anxiety Files. http://www.psychologytoday.com/blog/anxiety-files/201002/social-anxiety-how-be-better-monkey

[16] Levenson, R. W. (1994). Human emotion: A functional view. I n P. Ekman & R.J. Davidson (Eds.), The nature of emotion: Fundamental questions (New York : Oxford University Press., 123.

[17] Mc Dougall, C. (2010). Born to Run: The Hidden Tribe, the Ultrarunners and the Greatest Race the World has Ever Se. en. London: Profile Books.

[18] Mac, Lean. P. D. (1990). The Triune Brain in Evolution. New York: Plenum Press.

[19] Mead, M. (1935). Sex and Temperament in Three Primitive Societies (1st ed.). New York: HarperCollins Publishers Inc.

[20] Mitchell, S. (2002). Bhagavad Gita: A New Translation. New York, Three Rivers Press.

[21] Nagy, N. (2012). The Egyptian revolution seen through the eyes of a psychiatrist. International Psychiatry, , 9, 62-64.

[22] Nesse, R. M., & Williams, G. C. (1994). Why we get sick. The new science of Darwinian medicine. New York: Times Books.

[23] Newman, J. D. (2002). Vocal communication and the triune brain. Physiology and Behavior , 79, 495-502.

[24] Ploog DW.(2003). The place of the Triune Brain in psychiatry. Physiology and Behavior, , 79, 487-493.

[25] Price, J. S. (2000). Subordination, self-esteem and depression. In Sloman, L. and Gilbert, P. (Eds.), Subord. ination and Defeat: An Evolutionary Approach to Mood Disorders and their Therapy. (Mahwah, NJ: Lawrence Erlbaum Associates., 165-177.

[26] Price, J. S. (2002). The triune brain, escalation de-escalation strategies and mood disorders. In: Cory GA Jr & Gardner R Jr (eds) The Evolutionary Neuroethology of Paul

MacLean: Convergences and Frontiers. Westport, CT: Praeger. 107-117. The text of this and some of my other papers can be read on my website: www.john-price.me.uk).

[27] Price, J. S. (2003). Evolutionary aspects of anxiety disorders. *Dialogues in Clinical Neuroscience*, 5, 223-236, http://www.ncbi.nlm.nih.gov/pmc/articles/PMC3181631/.

[28] Price, J. S., & Gardner Jr, R. (2009). Does submission to a deity relieve depression? Illustrations from the Book of Job and the Bhagavad Gita. Philosophical Papers and Reviews, July 2009 http://www.academicjournals.org/PPR/PDF/Pdf2009/July/Price%20and%20Gardner.pdf

[29] Risch, N., Herrell, R., Lehner, T., Liang, K., Eaves, L., Hoh, J., Griem, A., Kovacs, M., et al. (2009). Interaction between the serotonin transporter gene (5-HTTLPR), stressful life events, and risk of depression: a meta-analysis. Journal of the American Medical Association doi:10.1001/jama.2009.878.PMC 2938776. PMID 19531786. // www.pubmedcentral.nih.gov/articlerender.fcgi?tool=pmcentrez&artid=2938776., 301(23), 2462-2471.

[30] Sainsbury, M. J., & Price, J. S. (1962). Art and psychotherapy. Medical Journal of Australia, , 10, 196-198.

[31] Stone, M. H. (2002). History of anxiety disorders. In: Textbook of Anxiety Disorders eds. DJ Stein & E. Hollander. American Psychiatric Publishing, Washington, DC,, , 3-12.

[32] Tinbergen, N. (1963). On aims and methods of ethology. Zeitschrift fur Tierpsychologie. , 20, 410-433.

[33] Tira, K., Hakosalo, O., Kareinen, L., Thomas, A., Hiem-Björkman, A., Escriou, C., Arnold, P., & Lohi, H. Environmental effects on compulsive tail chasing in dogs. PLos One 7 (7): e4168, (2012). http://www.alphagalileo.org/ViewItem.aspx?ItemId=123268&CultureCode=en

[34] Troisi, A. (2005). The concept of alternative strategies and its relevance to psychiatry and clinical psychology. Neuroscience Biobehavioral Revue, , 29, 159-168.

[35] Watson, K. K., Ghodasra, J. H., & Platt, M. L. (2009). Serotonin transporter genotype modulates social reward and punishment in rhesus macaques. PLoS ONE 4(1): e4156. doi:10.1371/journal.pone.0004156

[36] Wilson, D. R., Price, J. S., & Preti, A. (2009). Critical learning periods for self-esteem: mechanisms of psychotherapy and implications for the choice between individual and group treatment. In GN Christodoulou, M Jorge, JE Mezzich (eds) Advances in Psychiatry, third volume. Athens: Beta Medical Publishers, , 75-81.

Section 2

Basic Research

Chapter 3

Searching for Biological Markers of Personality: Are There Neuroendocrine Markers of Anxiety?

Antonio Armario and Roser Nadal

Additional information is available at the end of the chapter

1. Introduction

1.1. Defining the concepts underlying differences in emotional reactivity

The existence of stable individual differences in cognitive and emotional capabilities both in animals and humans is well-accepted. The theories of personality assume that such individual differences can be categorized and that the richness of individual differences in humans would be the result of the combination of differences in a few underlying personality factors. The most accepted contemporary theory is that of "Big Five" [1] that consider five highest order factors: neuroticism, extraversion, openness, agreeableness and conscientiousness. However, the nature of some of the putative factors is still a matter of dispute in the different theories. Within this framework, the factors extraversion and neuroticism have been associated to the response to positive and negative emotions, respectively. Moreover, it is typically distinguished between personality and temperament, the latter term referring to biological predisposition that is noted early in life and will eventually lead to adult personality [2]. Emotionality may be considered as relatively stable individual characteristic so that subjects labeled as highly emotional will strongly react to emotional stimuli, particularly negative ones. It is of interest to know how high neuroticism subjects react to stressful situations and which are the consequences of such exposure. It has been reported that in response to an adverse event high neuroticism soldiers showed larger increases in psychiatric symptoms than low neuroticism subjects [3], but no differences in the response were observed after controlling for pre-trauma symptoms. These data question the existence of high stress responsiveness in high neuroticism subjects.

In animals, the concept of emotionality is associated with the response to aversive stimuli. On the basis of the study of the behavioral and physiological responses to emotional situations, it may be concluded that emotional reactivity is clearly multifactorial. For instance, neither behavioral nor physiological responses, all of them presumably related to this concept, follow a uniform pattern when different strains of rats are compared [4]. The obvious conclusion is that emotionality is a complex, multifactorial, concept [4] and that emotional stimuli are probably processed in parallel brain circuits thus resulting in a wide range of associated physiological responses.

For the purpose of the present review we will focus on individual differences in anxiety. This is a particular emotional characteristic that has attracted considerable attention for the important role of anxiety disorders in humans. It is generally distinguished between the concepts of trait and state anxiety. The first refers to a stable predisposition to react with low or high levels of anxiety in response to anxiety-provoking stimuli, whereas the second evaluate the actual reaction to a particular situation. Some classical psychometric test distinguish between both, for instance the trait-state anxiety Spielberger test or STAI [5], trait anxiety being a general predisposition to get higher levels of state anxiety when confronted with aversive situations. The distinction between trait and state anxiety is particularly difficult in animal models, although some authors assumed, in line with the concept in humans, that animals characterized by high levels of trait anxiety should show high levels of anxiety-like behaviour in response to different tests, as it is the case of BALB/c inbred mice [6]. There is no consensus about putative tests that can specifically evaluate differences in trait anxiety in animals. Another important theoretical consideration is the distinction between normal and pathological anxiety, the latter one reflecting merely the extreme of a continuum, or on the contrary qualitative differences with the normal population. This distinction is basically impossible to establish in animal models.

When discussing about animal models, it is important to distinguish between those that involve certain environmental or genetic manipulations aimed to develop high anxious individuals or those aiming at evaluating anxiety-like behaviour in particular individuals. We referred to the latter as tests for anxiety or anxiety-like behaviour. There are different animal tests for anxiety. Some of them involve unconditioned response to aversive stimuli, whereas others imply conditioned responses [6]. Even when unconditioned tests, which usually involve evaluation of the free behaviour of animals, are used there are many instances of dissociation in the outcomes of the different tests when comparing groups of animals [i.e. 7]. This suggests that each test probably evaluate situational-specific components of anxiety. In fact, factorial analysis sometimes supports that putatively underlying factors determining behaviour are likely to differ in great part across tests [i.e. 8,9]. This is important when considering the putative relationship between anxiety and physiological parameters to be discussed later. Nevertheless, marked differences in trait-anxiety, either of environmental or genetic origin, may result in important differences in several different behavioral tests [i.e. 10,11], suggesting partially common underlying factors.

It is now widely-accepted that there are conceptual differences between fear and anxiety in that fear is elicited by precise and temporally defined dangers (the presence of a predator, exposure to well-announced aversive stimuli such as electric shocks), whereas anxiety would be elicited by more diffuse and sustained dangers (contextual fear conditioning, predator odours, unpredictable aversive stimuli) [12, 13]. Nevertheless, it is still difficult to be sure whether behaviour of animals in novel environments is related to fear or anxiety. For instance, rats and mice have innate aversion for open spaces, likely to be related to the risks of being predated in such places. Can then we speak about fear (innate predisposition) or about anxiety so far as the open spaces is only potentially nor actually dangerous? This is important as several widely used anxiety tests are based on exposure to novel environments such as the elevated plus-maze (EPM) or the light-dark (or dark-light) tests [14-17]. The EPM consists of a plus-maze elevated over the floor, with two (closed) arms surrounded by walls and other two unprotected. The light-dark apparatus has two compartments, one small and dark and another much greater and illuminated. In the light-dark version we initially put the animals into the illuminated area and measure time spent to entry for the first time in the dark compartment, the number of transitions between light and dark and the time spent in each compartment. In the dark-light version, the animals are introduced into the dark compartment and we measure the latency to enter into the illuminated area and the other measures previously indicated. The EPM and light-dark test are based on the fear elicited in rodents (which are nocturnal animals) by open and illuminated spaces, and the natural tendency of these animals to explore new environments. These two tendencies generated a conflict and we expect that less emotional, fearless or low anxiety animals spend more time in the open arms of the EPM and the illuminated area of the light-dark test. Other animal models are based on the performance in an active avoidance-escape task in a shuttle box. In this task the imminence of a shock is signalled by a specific conditioned stimulus (noise, light; CS) and the animals can learn to avoid the shock (during the CS) or escape from the actual shock by doing a particular active behaviour: jumping from one side to the other. This procedure likely elicits an emotional reaction close to fear. However poor performance in such task is considered to be associated to high anxiety that makes the animals to become immobile and perform poorly. Administration of classical anxiolytic drugs clearly improves performance [i.e. 18]. The extent to which psychological dimensions underlying individual differences are similar in all cases or whether or not we are really detecting differences in anxiety is still an open question.

In addition to the problem of correctly indentifying a particular behavioral trait, there are problems related to the characterization of the physiological profiles associated to such a trait. First, negative emotional situations elicit a wide range of physiological responses and it is important to know whether or not such repertoire of responses is dependent of the particular stimulus or the particular emotion elicited. Until now it has not been possible to conclusively identify physiological response patterns associated to specific emotions. Second, the emotional response to particular situations are greatly influenced by the cognitive processing of the particular stimulus (appraisal) and by coping strategies, that is the behavioral repertoire used for the animals to escape from the source of the aversive experience or to reduce the impact of the situation. Koolhaas [19] considered coping style as a set of coherent behavioral and physiological responses to aversive stimuli. Two different coping styles have been defined: proactive (active) and reactive (passive), characterized by the triggering of active versus passive strategies to cope with aversive situations. The authors considered coping style as independent of emotionality [19,20]. That is, the dimension of active *versus* passive strategies is considered as orthogonal to emotionality. Nevertheless, coping style can influence the success of the strategy used to face the situation and, indirectly, the behavioral and physiological response to the situation. Therefore, it is difficult to establish putative relationship between physiological variables and emotionality, including anxiety, without knowing other dimensions of personality as coping style.

It should be also taken into account that even if we can isolate one particular trait such as anxiety, the final behavioral and physiological responses (measurable outputs) are the result of the activation (or inhibition) of a wide range of divergent brain pathways, each of them putatively influenced by individual characteristics not related to the trait of interest, which may perturb or mask the common influence (trait) on all these variables. For instance, if we evaluate emotional reactivity by the activity of animals in a novel environment, even if two animals experienced the same level of fear/anxiety, the expression of the final measured response (ambulation, rearing) could differ because of different in activity, coping strategies (active or passive) or other traits (i.e. interest for novelty). Available evidence indicates that the genetic control of anxiety appears to be polygenic (as it is the case of other behavioral traits). Similar conclusion applies to the control of certain physiological parameters important for the present issue, as it is the case of the hypothalamic-pituitary-adrenal (HPA) axis [21]. By definition, inbred rats are genetically homogeneous and homozygotic for all genes. This means that every inbred strain has only a particular allele for each gene among the various ones present in the species and that throughout the process of inbreeding, a particular allele of each gene involved in the behavioral trait of interest or in the activity of the HPA axis has been randomly fixed. As it can be assumed that the genes are controlling each particular function in both positive and negative directions, each particular inbred strain could have been fixed a different combination of the alleles involved in the functions of interest. Therefore, it may be theoretically difficult to find a relationship between a behavioral trait and the HPA axis that may apply to other inbred strains or to an outbred population of rats. That is why we will refer only in very specific cases to studies with inbred rats or mice.

1.2. An overview of the HPA axis and other physiological stress markers

The present review will focus on the relationship between anxiety and the sympathetic-medullo-adrenal (SMA) and hypothalamic-pituitary endocrine axes. In the latter case, special attention should be given to the HPA axis and prolactin because they are considered as good biological markers of stress (see below). Activation of the SMA and HPA axes constitute the prototypical physiological responses to stressors in all vertebrates. These two axes have focused great attention in the field of stress for two main reasons [22]. First, the release of SMA and HPA hormones into blood is positively related to the intensity of the stressful situations and therefore they are well-suited to reflect differences among subjects in the degree of emotional activation. Second, activation of the SMA axis have a critical role in the regulation of metabolism and cardiovascular responses and is likely to be important for the development of certain stress-related pathologies (i.e. hypertension). Third, glucocorticoids (cortisol in humans and most mammals; corticosterone in rats and mice), the final output hormone of the HPA axis, has been implicated in a wide range of pathophysiological and psychopathological processes, including cardiovascular diseases, immune suppression, altered gastrointestinal function, anxiety disorders, depression and predisposition to drug self-administration. However, It is now well-recognized that stress-induced pathology is not only dependent on the nature and time-schedule of exposure to stressors but on individual differences in vulnerability to them.

The association between the activation of the SMA axis and stress is well-known since the earlier works by Cannon in the first half of the XX century. However, it is now realized that stress exposure also resulted in the activation of certain responses mediated by the parasympathetic nervous system. For instance, changes in intestinal colonic motility and visceral pain sensitivity [i.e. 23-25]. Moreover, the old idea that the SMA axis is activated in an all or none manner is not accepted as there are strong anatomical and functional evidence for a fine tuning of the response of SMA to different stimuli, including stressors [26, 27]. The flexibility of the SMA axis to respond to different stimuli is on the basis of the theories that argue that different emotions in humans can be distinguished by a particular physiological signature, nevertheless, there is not at present unequivocal and precise evidence for such signature [28]. Activation of the SMA axis have been typically evaluated measuring plasma (or urinary) levels of noradrenaline and adrenaline, heart rate (HR), heart rate variability (HRV, a measure of parasympathetic cardiac activity), diastolic and systolic blood pressure (DBP; SBP) and electric skin conductance. Plasma levels of adrenaline derived almost totally from the adrenal medulla, whereas plasma noradrenaline derived in part from the adrenal medulla but mostly from the activity of sympathetic nerves in all body. It is well-established that both plasma adrenaline and noradrenaline increases in response to emotional stressors, but the former better reflects the intensity of emotional stressors [29]. As circulating adrenaline is the main factor controlling stress-induced hyperglycaemia, it is not surprising that plasma glucose is a marker of stress intensity under moderate to strong stressful conditions [29].

The HPA axis is a complex and dynamic system whose regulation has been very well-characterized in the last decades [30]. The main brain locus of control of the HPA axis is the paraventricular nucleus of the hypothalamus (PVN). The PVN is a complex nucleus with two main types of neurons and several subdivisions. Big (magnocellular) neurons are located in the PVNm and synthesize the neurohypophyseal hormones oxytocin and vasopressin (VP), sending axons directly to the neurohypophysis. Small (parvocellular) neurons are concentrated in the PVNp and send axons to the median eminence to release ACTH secretagogues into the pituitary portal blood. Among such secretagogues, the corticotropin releasing factor (hormone) (CRF or CRH) is considered to be the most important in that it controls both synthesis and release of the adrenocorticotropic hormone (ACTH) and other peptides derived from pro-opiomelanocortin (POMC) in anterior pituitary corticotrope cells. Among the other ACTH secretagogues, VP appears to play a prominent role, acting synergistically with CRH to increase the release (but not the synthesis) of ACTH. In the PVNp appears to be two different populations of CRH neurons, one co-expressing and another one non-coexpressing VP. Interestingly, persistent or repeated activation of the HPA axis is accompanied by an increase in the number of CRH neurons coexpressing VP in the PVNp, suggesting a more prominent role of VP in those situations associated to hyperactivity of the HPA axis. CRH in the anterior pituitary acts through CRH type 1 receptors (CRH-R1), whereas VP acts through AVP1b receptors. In addition to the above considerations, it should be taken into account that the contribution of CRF, VP and other secretagogues to the release of HPA hormones appears to be dependent on the particular type of stressor.

When the animals are exposed to stressful situations ACTH is promptly released (a few minutes), reaching a maximum between 5-10 minutes after a brief exposure to stressors or between 15-30 minutes with more prolonged exposures. Plasma levels of ACTH may well reflect a wide range of stressor intensities provided that samples are taken at appropriate times after the initial exposure to the stressor [29]. If exposure to a stressor lasts only a few minutes, maximal ACTH levels are achieved in a period of 5-10 minutes, then declining. If exposure to the stressor continues and it is relatively severe, the ACTH response is maintained for about 1 h but not more, and, therefore, plasma levels of ACTH are no longer a reflection of stressor intensity. One critical point regarding stress-induced adrenocortical secretion is that the maximum is reached with relatively low levels of ACTH so that plasma levels of glucocorticoids are only a good reflection of ACTH release with low intensity stressors. In fact, differences in plasma levels of corticosterone immediately after exposure to relatively severe stressors (i.e. footshock, restraint, immobilization) reflect more the maximal capability of the adrenal to secrete glucocorticoids, which is related to the adrenal weight [i.e. 31], rather than the circulating levels of ACTH, thus leading to a frequent misinterpretation of the results.

On the basis of the above, two major points should be considered in evaluating the impact of a stressor on the HPA axis. Firstly, measurement of circulating levels of glucocorticoids at a time shorter than 15 minutes after initial exposure to stress is non-appropriate to reflect the actual impact of a stressor on adrenocortical secretion because maximum levels are achieved nearly and beyond this time point. Secondly, plasma levels of glucocorticoids are not a reflection of stressor intensity above a certain level of intensity, which usually lies within low to moderate range. In the rat, exposure to a relatively stressful novel environment is probably the situation above which glucocorticoids hardly can detect actual anterior pituitary activation. Although, plasma glucocorticoids levels just after stress did not reflect ACTH levels, the follow-up of their plasma levels for a period of time after the termination of stress can reflect the initial ACTH release and therefore should be used in those cases where there is no possibility to directly measure ACTH.

Glucocorticoids release by stress exerts a wide range of actions in the body, both peripherally and centrally. These effects are exerted through genomic and non-genomic processes [32, 33]. Genomic effects of glucocorticoids are exerted through two well-characterized receptors: mineralocorticoid (MR, type I) and glucocorticoid (GR, type II) receptors. The non-genomic receptors are still uncharacterized at the molecular level, but are likely to be located in plasmatic membrane. Regarding the regulation of the HPA axis, one major function of glucocorticoids is to exert a negative feedback to reduce initial activation of the HPA axis. This negative feedback [34] is exerted at different levels: at the anterior pituitary, at the PVN and at other key brain areas such as the hippocampal formation and the prefrontal cortex

[30]. The negative glucocorticoid feedback controls both normal resting activity of the HPA axis and the response to stressors. Since a defective negative feedback can markedly alter HPA functioning, there are classical tests for the efficacy of such feedback that use exogenous administration of natural or synthetid glucorticoids. In humans, it is extensively used the administration of the synthetic glucocorticoid dexamethasone (DEX) in the so called suppression DEX test. However, the validity of this test has been questioned by the fact that DEX, which easily penetrated the brain, is excluded from the brain by the multi-drug resistant protein P-glycoprotein [35]. Therefore, depending on the dose DEX mainly acts at the pituitary and only to a limited extent within the brain.

The HPA axis shows both circadian and pulsatile rhythms [36]. In addition to its biological meaning, the existence of a pulsatile secretion of ACTH and corticosterone is an important concern when only one sample is taken as it could not be representative of the actual secretion. Regarding circadian rhythm, maximum activity is observed around the awakening time. Maximum levels of plasma glucocorticoids are associated in all animals and humans to the start of the active period, being observed just around lights off in rats and mice and just after sleep in humans. Although the circadian rhythm affects both ACTH and glucocorticoids, the amplitude is much greater for the latter than for ACTH due to an increase in adrenal sensitivity to circulating ACTH [37]. In humans, there is a sharp increase in the first 30 minutes after awakening (called the cortisol awakening response, CAR) followed by a progressive decline over the day [38, 39]. Both in animals and humans, proper evaluation of the HPA axis requires taking several samples over the day.

Measurement of plasma levels of ACTH and corticosterone under resting (basal) conditions and after exposure to stress is the simplest approach when studying the functionality of the HPA axis. It is important to note that altered responsiveness of HPA hormones to stress can be observed with normal resting levels, but increased responsiveness to stressors may eventually result in increased resting levels of plasma glucocorticoids. However, these measures are very often insufficient for a deeper understanding of HPA differences between individuals or between different physiological or pathological conditions. Other classical measures include the evaluation of: (a) adrenal responsiveness to ACTH by administering exogenous ACTH and measuring plasma levels of cortisol or corticosterone; (b) adrenocorticotrope cell responsiveness to CRH and VP by exogenous administration of these neurohormones and measurement of plasma levels of glucocorticoids and preferable of ACTH; (c) the integrity of negative glucocorticoid feedback mechanisms, usually by given DEX. More recently, the combined DEX-CRH test has gained considerable interest, although the biological processes underlying this test are not well-understood. In animals, we can obviously use a wide range of additional approaches, but the most used are the evaluation of the brain expression of those neuropeptides directly related to the regulation of the HPA axis. If some subjects respond more to stress, it is assumed that they will ideally show enhanced PVN expression of CRH and/or VP, enhanced AP expression of the POMC gene, increased adrenal weight and perhaps higher resting levels of plasma glucocorticoids and reduced efficacy of negative glucocorticoid feedback. This is a typical pattern after exposure of animals to chronic severe stressors [40]; however, it is realistic to assume that this whole pattern would be rarely found in humans.

Individual differences in some of the components of this complex biological system may oppose to the expected results, complicating the interpretation of the results. For instance, a highly emotional rat or mouse strain may be characterized by a physiological defect in the HPA axis (i.e. defective CRH production, reduced adrenocortical responsiveness to ACTH) that would act in the opposite direction to emotionality thus cancelling the differences in particular hormonal output. This is the case of inbred Lewis rats. They are considered as highly emotional [4], but are also characterized by a defective HPA system thus resulting in reduced ACTH and corticosterone response to a wide range of stressors (i.e. 41, 42). Therefore, if we expect higher HPA activation in these emotional animals (a hypothesis that is not necessarily true), defective HPA function could mask the expected higher HPA response. This problem is particularly important when comparing inbred animals.

In addition to the HPA axis, all anterior pituitary hormones (growth hormone, GH, thyrotropin stimulating hormone, TSH, prolactin, luteinizing hormone, LH, and follicle-stimulating hormone, FSH) have been extensively studied regarding stress and psychopathology. However, in recent decades, the interest focused on the HPA axis and to lower extent in prolactin. Prolactin is a stress-responsive hormone that is regulated by two hypothalamic mechanisms [43]. One involves a potent and tonic inhibitory control by a population of dopaminergic neurons located in the arcuate nucleus that send axons to the pituitary portal blood (tuberoinfundibular system). The other involves one or several prolactin releasing factors (PRFs). There are several candidates as PRFs, including oxytocin and VP, but there is no still agreement about the actual PRF. It is likely that during stress, prolactin release is the consequence of the reduction of dopaminergic inhibitory signals and the increase in stimulatory inputs. Although the precise role of prolactin during stress is not known, there is evidence that peripheral prolactin has access to the brain through prolactin receptors and can exert anxiolytic and anti-stress effects [44].

1.3. Are the intensity and nature of the stressor important for characterizing individual differences?

Which are the objectives of characterizing individual differences in responsiveness to stressors? One important purpose is to associate altered physiological responsiveness to pathological conditions: i.e., increased cortisol response to stressors may underlie immune suppression. Another one is to establish whether or not certain individuals or psychopathologies are characterized by an altered sensitivity to stressors. In the latter case, we assume that the chosen physiological variable is able to distinguish between hypo- or hyper-responsive subjects. However, to accomplish this goal we need to demonstrate first that these variables are able to reflect the intensity of stressors and that the results are relatively unaffected by the type (quality) of stressor. In animals, on the basis of neuronal activation as revealed by c-fos and lesion experiments it appears that those stressors having a predominant emotional component (i.e. electric shock, restraint, immobilization, exposure to predator or predator odors) activate the HPA axis following telencephalic pathways, whereas stressors having a predominantly physical component (endotoxin, cytokines, hemorrhage) act primarly at the level of the brainstem, brainstem nuclei sending stimulatory signals to the PVNp [45, 46]. In fact, recent studies suggest that is likely that each particular stressor can have a particular brain activation signature, thus leading to differential adaptive behavioral and physiological responses and pathological consequences [47]. Nevertheless, it has been demonstrated in rats and mice that in response to predominantly emotional stressors, plasma levels of adrenaline, noradrenaline, ACTH, corticosterone (under certain conditions) and prolactin reflect, under appropriate conditions, the intensity of stressors [29]. In contrast, whereas circulating levels of some other anterior pituitary hormones (GH, TSH, LH) are altered by stress in animals and humans [i.e. 48-51], there is no evidence that they are sensitive to the intensity of stressors. In rats, we have found a very consistent correlation between the ACTH or corticosterone response to different novel environments [52, 53], whereas no correlation at all when comparing the response to a novel environment and to a much more severe stressor such as immobilization (unpublished). Whether or not the critical factor for the lost of correlation is the markedly different intensity of the two stressors or the qualitative differences among them is unclear.

In humans, despite the extensive human literature on stress, there have been few attempts to establish which physiological variables may be sensitive to the intensity of emotional stressors. Callister [54] used two tests (a modified Stroop colour word test and mental arithmetic task) each with different levels of difficulty over one unique session and observed progressive increases in the perceived stress in function of the difficulty; in contrast, HR was independent and DBP and SBP promptly achieved a plateau with relatively low levels of intensity. Therefore, there is negative evidence for a relationship between HR and level of stress and limited evidence regarding blood pressure. In our own work we compared in Medicine female students the anxiety, cortisol, prolactin and glucose responses to two exams (Psychology and Physiology) that were known to induce different levels of anxiety [55]. As expected, state anxiety increased in response to both exams as compared to a regular day, but anxiety was greater with Physiology. The response to plasma cortisol was low, but in the same direction, whereas prolactin not only increased with respect to the routine day, but the increase was greater with Physiology than Psychology exam. In another study, salivary cortisol appears to reflect the degree of stress when assessed in different situations during military survival training [56]. These data support the hypothesis that biological stress markers are likely to behave similarly in humans and rodents. Interestingly, despite the parallel behaviour of state anxiety, cortisol and prolactin, no significant correlation was observed between the variables in our work [55], suggesting parallel but in great part independent regulation. The Trier social stress test (TSST) is an extensively used psychosocial stress that includes public speech and evaluation [57]. Subjects classified as high or low responders in function of the ACTH and cortisol responses to the TSST did not differ in their HR, adrenaline or noradrenaline responses [58]. This suggests that classification of subjects was based more on a specific functional difference in the regulation of the HPA or on individual differences in stress responsiveness that only affected the HPA axis, not reflecting a general stress hyper-responsiveness.

In sum, the available results are not suggestive of a stressor-independent pattern of response of the HPA axis and other variables that could unequivocally characterize individuals. That is, individual differences in physiological responsiveness to stressors are not only depending on certain characteristics of the individuals, but also on the particular stressor used as a challenge. Interestingly, attention should be paid as to how subjects can experience different emotional reactions to the same stressful situations. Thus, it was observed in healthy subjects a differential emotional response (evaluated by facial expression) to a mental arithmetic task that translated to a differential cardiovascular and salivary cortisol response [59]. In contrast, self-reported emotional experience did not contribute to such differential physiological response.

2. Neuroendocrinology of anxiety in humans

2.1. General considerations

In evaluating the neuroendocrinology of anxiety we can take some critical points into consideration. First, is there any relationship between state anxiety and certain hormones in response to some acute aversive situations? Second, is there any relationship between trait anxiety in a non-pathological population and resting or stress levels of hormones? Third, are resting or stress levels of hormones altered in pathological anxiety?

It is well-known in humans that exposure to acute stress can induce physiological (including hormonal) changes and increased anxiety, with a pattern quite similar to that observed in animals. However, there are numerous inconsistencies in the literature regarding the response of cortisol or prolactin to stressors. This is likely to be due to our poor knowledge on the dose-response relationship between stressor intensity and the elicited physiological and anxious responses in humans. The characterization of the dose-response curves of stressor intensity and physiological variables is critical for three main reasons. First, we can identify which physiological variables are actually sensitive to the intensity of stressors, thus ruling out those which are not. Second, we need to know which range of intensity of stressors can be appropriately evaluated using a particular variable. For instance, we know that in rodents plasma corticosterone is useful for low to intermediate intensity stressors but not for the intermediate-severe intensities, whereas the opposite is true for plasma glucose. Third, if the physiological response is well-characterized, this can help to objectively place any experimental stressful situation within the stress scale. Finally, and importantly, if we are using experimental situations eliciting a modest (or a very high) physiological response, the characterization of individual differences should be theoretically more difficult. This is particularly critical when the experimental conditions only elicited an extremely low, if any, response as appear to be the case in an important number of papers [for review, see 60].

In analyzing the literature about individual differences in responsiveness to stressful laboratory tasks, it is important to consider the importance of pre-task hormone levels. It has been repeatedly observed that some physiological markers of stress are elevated by the anticipation of the task rather than by the task itself. This sometimes leads to misinterpretation of the results as a reduced response to the task. In fact, anticipatory anxiety and physiological response may be indicative of high rather than reduced responsiveness to putative stressful situations.

2.2. Neuroendocrinology of anxiety in healthy subjects

Unless otherwise stated, differences in trait or state anxiety were evaluated with the well-characterized STAI. We will comment first data regarding state anxiety and then trait anxiety.

Although numerous studies have demonstrated increases in both state anxiety and some physiological parameters in response to stressful situations, only few studies reported correlation between them. In an important number of studies correlation between state anxiety and some hormones was low or absent, suggesting that despite the apparent parallelism, underlying factors are likely to differ. In response to anticipation of surgery a significant correlation was observed between state anxiety and cortisol, but not prolactin [61]. In contrast, no association between anxiety and the increases in cortisol, prolactin or TSH levels were observed after parachute jumping [50]. In our own work with exam stress, no significant correlation was found between state STAI anxiety and plasma cortisol or prolactin levels [55]. Similarly, in a speech task, some correlations were found between certain physiological parameters (HR, BP, noradrenaline, cortisol), but not between them and state anxiety [62]. Pottier et al [63] observed in medical students that consultation in an unfamiliar ambulatory setting caused more anxiety (as evaluated by the STAI and a visual analog scale, VAS) and salivary cortisol response than consultation in a familiar (in-hospital) setting, but no correlation was found between the two measures. Similarly, VAS anxiety did not appear to predict changes in cortisol or HR response to the TSST test in young males whereas perceived stress did [64]. A study with arithmetic stress observed significant correlation between state anxiety and salivary α-amylase, but not cortisol or chromogranin-A [65]. Salivary α-amylase and chromogranin-A both reflect SMA activation, but it is possible that salivary α-amylase represents a specific component of SMA activation more closely related to anxiety than other SMA markers and cortisol. In contrast to most of the previous results, a study evaluating in surgeons the physiological and STAI response to 54 different surgical procedures (some of them not perceived as stressful) observed significant correlations between STAI and HR or salivary cortisol, and between HR and cortisol [66].

In conclusion, the above results did not reveal a consistent positive relationship between state anxiety and physiological response to stressors. One theoretical explanation for the inconsistencies may be explained by the type of data incorporated to the measurement of correlation. If we include data corresponding to different stressful situations differing in intensity and, therefore, in the magnitude of the response of certain variables (i.e. anxiety and cortisol), obviously both variables would increase in parallel. Consequently, a positive correlation should be observed (Fig. 1). In contrast, if we consider only the same data corresponding to each particular stressful situation, no correlation could be observed. In addition, there are other possibilities to explain this lack of consistent relationship. Firstly, failure to find association may be due to methodological problems such as the clearly different dynamics of each variable that make it very difficult to design experiments optimizing all variables. Secondly, physiological variables may capture specific psychological processes, only some of them being more specifically related to measures of anxiety. Finally, dissociation may exist between subjective and physiological measures of emotion. For instance, invasive cardiologists showed increased anxiety response when they adopted a secondary assistant (teaching) than a primary operator (autonomous) role, but this subjective state was not associated to higher HR and salivary cortisol responses [67].

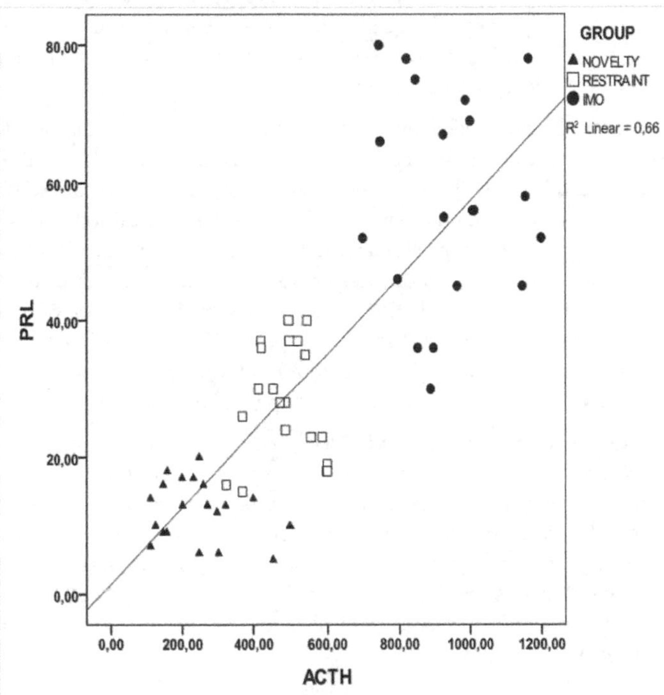

Figure 1. Correlation between two physiological measures (ACTH and prolactin, PRL) in a simulated response to three stressors of different intensity: a novel environment, restraint in tubes, and immobilization on boards (IMO). It should be noticed than when all samples are considered there is a positive statistical significant correlation between the two hormones, whereas no correlation at all was found when only samples corresponding to the same stressor were studied. This can explain inconsistencies in the literature regarding correlations between physiological variables and between them and state anxiety.

Regarding trait anxiety, there is negative evidence for an association between trait anxiety and salivary cortisol response to a speech task or the TSST in adult males [68. 69]. In a study that compared the response to the TSST of controls and patients with chronic atopic disease, the lack of relationship between trait-anxiety and salivary cortisol was confirmed and extended to plasma levels of ACTH [70]. Similarly, no relationship was found between trai and state anxiety and salivary amylase and cortisol responses to TSST or electrical stimulation either in males or females [71]. Surprisingly, some authors have reported a negative rather than positive relationship between trait anxiety and stress responsiveness. Healthy subjects classified as highly anxious showed a diminished salivary cortisol response to an unpleasant film as compared to low anxiety subjects [72]. This result has been extended in two studies showing lower plasma ACTH, cortisol, prolactin, adrenaline and noradrenaline in response to psychosocial stress (public speech) in anxious versus non-anxious subjects [73, 74]. Moreover, similar results were obtained using the Hospital Anxiety and Depression Scale that evaluated BP, HR and salivary cortisol responses to a combined (Stroop test, mirror-tracing and speech) psychosocial stressor [75]. The above data thus suggest a negative rather than positive relationship between neuroendocrine markers and trait anxiety, although neurobiological underpinnings are unknown.

The relationship between trait anxiety and resting activity of the HPA axis has also attracted attention. There is no association with basal salivary evening cortisol [76] or the cortisol response to the DEX+CRH test [77]. However, trait anxiety appears to affect the circadian rhythm of salivary cortisol in military men under free-living conditions, those with high trait anxiety displaying less pronounced decreased from early morning to mid-morning [78]. In post-pubertal adolescents, high trait anxiety resulted in higher evening salivary cortisol with no differences in morning levels [79]. Taken together, trait anxiety may be associated to a dysregulation of circadian resting cortisol levels, particularly the decline over the waking period, although there are discrepancies in the details. Studies measuring ACTH are needed to discern between ACTH-dependent or ACTH-independent dysregulation.

Interestingly, in response to a stressful video (corneal transplant) where higher and faster increased was observed in saliva α-amylase than in cortisol, a significant positive correlation was observed between trait anxiety and α-amylase, but not cortisol [80]. A recent report in children exposed to 3 consecutive stressors (including performance and peer rejection) confirmed the positive relationship of trait anxiety (measured by the revised children's manifest anxiety scale) and baseline or stress levels of α-amylase [81]. Considering the previously discussed positive relationship between α-amylase and state anxiety, this parameter offers promising results in studies of anxiety.

2.3. Neuroendocrinology of anxiety disorders

The relationship between anxiety disorders and basal (non-stress) levels of classical stress hormones is not clear. There are different types of anxiety disorders, as defined by the DSM-IVR [82]: Panic attacks, agoraphobia, social phobia, obsessive-compulsive disorder, post-traumatic stress disorder and generalized anxiety disorder (GAD). We will focus mainly in GAD on this aspect as an example among the different anxiety disorders.

Measures of urinary cortisol give inconsistent results, whereas higher catecholamine content appears to be more consistent in patients (see review of earlier works in [83]). Plasma prolactin was found to be normal in early studies [83] and this was further confirmed [84]. Cerebrospinal fluid (CSF) levels of CRH are considered as an index of overall activity of brain CRH neurons, including those neuronal CRH populations not directly related to the regulation of the HPA axis. It appears that CSF CRH levels are not altered in GAD, suggesting normal brain CRH function [85]. In addition to the inconsistencies of early studies, data from some recent studies using salivary cortisol do not offer a clearer picture. In late-life GAD, increased resting levels of salivary cortisol were observed at several times in the morning but not the evening and the levels were positively related to the severity of anxiety [86]. In accordance, slightly higher awakening levels of cortisol were observed in a sample of patients with anxiety disorders, the effects being particularly significant in those with panic disorder with agoraphobia and those showing comorbidity with anxiety and depression [87]. In contrast, lower CAR was observed in another study with a large cohort of older adults with several types of anxiety disorders when compared to healthy controls [88]. No differences were observed at other times. Another study with middle-age people suffering from GAD showed no differences from controls either in the CAR or in the daily pattern of cortisol, despite higher levels of α-amylase [89]. Whether or not the inconsistencies are due to the age of patients or confounding factors is not known, although the latter concern should be taken into account considering the usually small magnitude of the effects. Quite interestingly, decreased levels of hair cortisol were recently observed in GAD patients despite no changes in salivary cortisol over the day under resting conditions [90]. As hair cortisol represents the integration of cortisol release over periods of months, the results support a negative relationship between GAD and HPA activity. It is unclear whether these patients show reduced response to daily stressors (and therefore, less release of cortisol) rather than reduced resting activity. This hypoactivity of the HPA axis does not appear to be a general characteristic of all anxiety disorders. Thus, slightly alterations in circadian and pulsatile secretion of cortisol and to a lesser extent in ACTH was reported in panic patients, with overall higher levels as compared to controls and increased amplitude of cortisol pulses [91].

Unfortunately, there are scarce studies on the comparison of the response to stress of GAD patients as compared to controls. In adolescents with GAD, increases in ACTH, GH and prolactin (but not noradrenaline, adrenaline and cortisol) were found in the phase of anticipation to the task in GAD patients but not in controls [92]. In contrast, no response to the task was observed.

Phobic subjects offer an interesting model for the study of the relationship between behavioral reaction to the situation and the concomitant physiological response. Severe anxiety was reported in patients with phobia to insects and small animals after forced exposure, whereas no changes were found in prolactin [93]. In a further study, increases in HR, blood pressure and plasma levels of adrenaline, noradrenaline, cortisol and GH were reported, although the increases in state anxiety were stronger and did not correlate to physiological responses [94]. The strong dissociation between subjective behavioral arousal and cortisol response to spider phobia was confirmed in another study comparing phobics and healthy controls [95]. Driving phobics as compared to controls showed increased anticipatory anxiety and cortisol response to driving, with further increases in anxiety but not cortisol during driving [96]. Moreover, no significant correlation was found between anxiety and cortisol in phobic subjects. Less clear is the response of social phobia patients to social stimuli. Salivary cortisol response to the TSST was similar in social phobic adolescent girls than in controls [97]. In contrast, in another study, children with social phobia showed greater trait anxiety (measured by the STAI for childrens, STAI-C) and also greater state anxiety and cortisol responses to a public speaking task than controls [98]. In the latter study, trait anxiety was positively related to cortisol, but it was not described whether both control and patients, which already differed in trait anxiety, were included in the same analysis. In children with social phobia, exposure to an adapted TSST resulted in higher baseline and TSTT-induced anxiety (scales for Iconic self-assessment of anxiety in children) than controls [99]. In physiological terms, baseline HR was higher and the response to the stressor lower in patients as compared to controls, whereas salivary cortisol and α-amylase response tended to be lower. Finally, a study comparing healthy controls, social phobia and post-traumatic stress (PTSD) patients showed higher salivary cortisol response to the TSST in social phobics as compared to controls and PTSD [100]. The authors also reported a positive correlation between cortisol response to the TSST and avoidance of angry faces in social phobics but not in controls. Taken together, all those data suggest at least a lower physiological than subjective response to the phobic situations.

Perhaps the strongest evidence for dissociation between subjective and physiological responses comes from patients with panic disorder. These patients have been studied during spontaneous panic attacks, after pharmacological provocation of panic attacks or in response to different types of stressors. During spontaneous attacks, despite strong subjective anxiety and physiological signs, changes in HR were not strong and changes in hormones (noradrenaline, adrenaline, GH and cortisol) were low and inconsistent, being the increases in prolactin the most consistent [83, 101]. When agoraphobic subjects were exposed to the phobic situation to trigger a panic attack, most of them experienced panic attacks while control subjects did not [102], but only the HR was higher in patients than in controls, whereas other measures (i.e. blood pressure, cortisol, prolactin or GH) did not differ. There are several pharmacological manipulations (i.e., lactate, CO2 inhalation, cholecistokinin-4, pentagastrin, doxapram or meta-chlorophenylpiperazine, m-CPP) that have been demonstrated to induce panic attacks only in a few healthy subjects, whereas they strongly induce panic attacks in almost all panic patients. This experimentally controlled approach has been extensively used to compare the physiological response (including GH, prolactin and cortisol) of panic patients and control subjects, but the results are difficult to interpret because of the effects of these manipulations on physiological variables. For instance, m-CPP is a serotoninergic drug that can pharmacologically induce the release of cortisol and GH. If the greater panicogenic effect of the drug on panic patients is paralleled by a greater cortisol and GH release [103], this can be interpreted as a parallelism between the subjective state and hormones, but also as a putative sensitization of brain serotoninergic pathways controlling these hormones in panic patients. Nevertheless, the overall conclusion is again that there are no parallelism between the strong anxiety- and panic-inducing effects of these manipulations in panic patients as compared to controls and the physiological response [104-111].

Finally, some studies aimed at characterizing the physiological response to stressors in panic patients. Fully remitted, medication-free panic patients exposed to a mild psychological stressor showed a clear anticipatory DBP response and a greater cortisol response to the stressor as compared to a normal population [112]. In another study, in response to public speaking, anticipatory anxiety developed in medication-free symptomatic patients as compared to normal subjects, whereas the anxiety response to the actual stressor was lower [113]. Salivary cortisol showed an anticipatory response, with no further response to the stressor [114], whereas a permanently higher (anticipatory) skin conductance was observed in patients that did not further respond at all to the stressor [113]. No differences were observed in HR, DBP and SBP. The anticipatory plasma or salivary cortisol responses were not detected in a study using the TSST as the stressor that nevertheless showed markedly reduced plasma and saliva cortisol responses in panic patients as compared to controls, associated to a normal HR response [115]. In a very recent report using mild shocks as the stressor, the anxiety and salivary cortisol and α-amylase response was studied in panic patients as compared to controls [116]. Then, patients were treated with the benzodiazepine anxiolytic alprazolam and classified as responder and non-responder to the therapy. When the two groups of patients and controls were retrospectively compared, it was found a similar anticipatory increase in anxiety in the two groups of patients as compared to controls, but an anticipatory increase in α-amylase (but not in cortisol), only in those panic patients who further responded to the therapy with alprazolam. The similar state anxiety response of responders and non-responders accompanied by a differential anticipatory cortisol and α-amylase response demonstrates again the dissociation between subjective and physiological measures.

Table 1 summarizes the relationship between anxiety and the neuroendocrine response to stressors in healthy people and with anxiety disorders. The experimental data indicate a lack of parallelism between subjective state or trait anxiety and neuroendocrine response to stressors in healthy subjects. In fact, there is some evidence for a negative relationship between trait anxiety and physiological response to stressors. Regarding anxiety disorders, a negative relationship is frequently observed in panic and GAD patients, and a lack of association in social phobia.

3. Emotionality, anxiety and neuroendocrine markers in selected rat lines

3.1. Selection on the basis of defecation rate: Maudsley reactive (MR) and Maudsley non-reactive (MRN) rats

The first genetic selection of a putative emotional strain of rats used the criterium of defecation rate in a novel, stressful, environment (an open-field) and led to the characterization of high defecation rate (MR) and low defecation (MRN) lines [see 117]. This selection also resulted in lower activity in the open-field of MR as compared to MNR rats, thus supporting the hypothesis that emotional animals would display a lower level of activity in a stressful, environment. However, it soon became evident that the relationship between defecation rate and activity in the open-field was more controversial than previously assumed and of much lower magnitude than that of defecation. In addition, not consistent differences have been observed in other anxiety test, including the EPM, the acoustic startle response (ASR), the light-dark test and the shock-induced conditioned suppression of appetitive operant task [118-121] perhaps related to the existence of two different stocks of rats (UK and USA). Unfortunately, there only two reports comparing the HPA response in the two strains: Abel et al [122] found no differences in plasma corticosterone levels after 10 minutes of exposure to an open-field or to forced swimming. However, Kosti et al. [123] observed greater ACTH response to restraint in MR vs MNR, despite no differences in plasma corticosterone. This apparent discrepancy is likely to be due to increased corticosterone responsiveness to ACTH in MNR. Therefore, MR and MNR, which differ in some aspects of emotionality but not clearly in anxiety-like behaviour, did appear to show differences in HPA function.

Population	**Physiological system**					
	SMA		**HPA**		**PRL**	
Healthy subjects						
State anxiety	≈ *		≈		≈	
Trait anxiety	≈ / ↓		≈ / ↓		≈ / ↓	
Anxiety disorders						
GAD	↓		A / ↓		A / ↓	
Phobia	phobic Ss	others	phobic Ss	others	phobic Ss	others
	↓	?	↓	?	↓	?
Social phobia	≈	?	≈	?	?	?
Panic	panic attack	others	panic attack	others	panic attack	others
	↓	A / ↓	↓	A / ↓	↓	?

≈ : no correlation or approximately normal response (* except α - amylase, see main text)

↓: reduced, at least with respect to subjective anxiety

A : anticipatory response

Ss: stimuli

? : not tested

PRL : prolactin

Table 1. Relationship between normal or pathological anxiety and physiological response to stress.

3.2. Selection on the basis of the EPM: high anxiety and low anxiety rats (HAB, LAB)

The only specific selection process aiming at selecting two strains of rats strongly differing in their performance in the EPM, the most widely used test for anxiety, has resulted in HAB and LAB rats, the former displaying very low levels of exploration of the open arms of the plus-maze [124]. In addition, HAB rats spent less time in light and make less number of transitions in a dark-light test, and also spent less time in the social interaction test [125], confirming differences in anxiety. It is important to note that HAB rats are less active in the forced swimming test [124, 126], a classical test to evaluate antidepressants [127], which presumably evaluates passive-active coping strategies [128]. Therefore, HAB rat appear to be prone to use passive coping strategies and to depression-like behavior.

HAB showed greater ACTH and corticosterone responses than LAB, mainly when the animals are forced to remain in the open arms (more stressful than the closed arms) of the EPM [129], but not when they can freely explore both open and closed arms [124]. Moreover, no differences were observed in the ACTH and corticosterone responses to forced swim, despite differences in behaviour [124]. Surprisingly, HAB rats showed lower ACTH response than LAB to social defeat [130], demonstrating that differences in responsiveness to stress was dependent on the particular type of stressor used. Therefore, extreme differences in anxiety, evaluated by the EPM, only resulted in consistent differences in the HPA response to situations similar to those that serves as criteria for selection. When exposed to other situations, the results can markedly change. These data are very important because they suggest that individual differences in HPA responsiveness to stress are critically dependent on the type of stressor used.

HAB-LAB rats likely represent the most complete characterization of genetic differences in the HPA axis. In several reports it has been demonstrated enhanced VP gene expression in the PVN, affecting both magnocellular and parvocellular subdivisions [131]. In another report, enhanced PVN CRH expression was also observed [132]. These data suggest increased drive to the corticotrope cells, what is supported by an enhanced POMC gene expression in the anterior pituitary [133]. No differences were observed in CRH-R1 in the anterior pituitary, whereas there were increases in CRH-R2 (the other type of CRH receptor) and V1b receptors in the HAB rats [134]. It is quite possible that VP is responsible for the enhanced ACTH response to the DEX+CRH test in HAB rats [131], as the ACTH response to the mere administration of exogenous CRH was normal [135] and there are no differences between lines in the expression of GR in the anterior pituitary [131, 133]. Although most of the above described changes in the central aspects of the HPA axis may be better ascribed to depression-like rather than anxiety-like behavior, administration of an VP receptor antagonist in the PVN normalize anxiety-like behaviour of HAB rats [134]. This strongly suggests that enhanced PVN VP expression plays a critical role in anxiety.

The data regarding the PVN and the anterior pituitary would suggest increased drive to the gland and a generalized greater ACTH response to stress in HAB rats. However, this is not the case as reported above. A greater adrenal gland is associated in a normal population of rats with greater maximal corticosterone secretion [31]. Therefore, the increased adrenal cortex size of HAB rats is compatible with a greater maximal corticosterone secretion. In fact, HAB rats showed a normal ACTH response to endotoxin accompanied by a greater corticosterone response [136], which is likely to be maximal secretion under these conditions.

3.3. Selection on the basis of active avoidance performance

Several pairs of rat lines have been obtained on the basis of performance in passive or active avoidance tasks in a shuttle-box, using electric footshock as the aversive stimulus. Some, but not all, of these strains appears to differ in emotionality, particularly in fear/anxiety, but is should be taken into account that even if they actually differed in anxiety, also could differ in other traits (i.e. novelty-seeking or depression like behavior) that may affect the neuroendocrine response. These caveats should be taken into consideration in the discussion that follows.

The outbred Roman high avoidance (RHA) and Roman low avoidance (RLA) rats were obtained by genetic selection on the basis of performance in a two-way active avoidance task [see 20]. Most of the behavioral and endocrinological studies have been obtained in different substocks of the swiss sublines (RHA/Verh, RLA/Verh) and later by inbred RHA and RLA strains. It was soon realized that the two lines differed not only in active avoidance, but also in terms of emotionality, the RLA rats being more emotional than RHA rats. Subsequent research has demonstrated that the two lines differ in several important behavioral traits, including coping style and impulsivity [20]. The lines differ in some tests of anxiety more markedly than in others, being particularly relevant the inconsistencies regarding the EPM [137].

There have been some discrepancies regarding the responsiveness of the HPA axis to stress in these strains. In 1982, Gentsch et al. [138] firstly reported that RHA/Verh rats showed lower ACTH, corticosterone and prolactin responses to mild stressors (i.e. novel environments) than RLA/Verh rats, but the differences disappeared with stronger (i.e. ether stress, footshock, restraint) stressors. However, inconsistent differences were observed in when the lines were maintained in another laboratory [139, 140]. The study by Walker et al [141] is one of the most complete characterizations of differences in the HPA axis between the two lines. Unfortunately, the results are extremely difficult to interpret. Thus, it was found in RHA as compared to RLA rats: (a) higher adrenal weight; (b) higher basal levels of ACTH accompanied by normal corticosterone levels; (c) no differences in ACTH levels after 10 minutes of exposure to a novel environment or ether (10 minutes), despite an enhanced anterior pituitary response to exogenous CRH administration; (c) a lower corticosterone response to stressor despite the normal levels of ACTH and the increased adrenal weight. In addition, a higher number of GR in the pituitary along with higher MR levels in the hippocampus was found in RHA rats. The higher number of GR in the anterior pituitary may have contributed to the reduced ACTH response to CRH, whereas the higher MR in the hippocampus could be expected, if any, to reduce ACTH response to stress, which was not the case (in absolute terms) in their paper. In further reports, the early findings of increased ACTH and corticosterone responsiveness of RLA rats to novel environments were confirmed [137, 142]. Moreover, RLA rats showed normal levels of CRF mRNA, but increased levels of VP mRNA in the PVNp [142], a pattern observed in situations characterized by a chronic hyperactivity of the HPA axis. At first glance, the latter results suggest that HPA axis of RLA may be generally more responsive to stress than RHA, thus resulting in increased VP gene expression in the PVN. However, one could expect a greater relative adrenal weight in RLA as a consequence of the cumulative impact of higher ACTH response to daily events, but the opposite has been repeatedly found [139, 141, 143]. The possibility remains that the greater adrenal weight of RHA vs RLA rats is a compensatory mechanisms to maintain appropriate adrenocortical secretion despite some defect at the level of the adrenal.

Genetic analysis of cosegregation of different behavioral and physiological variables in these lines has allowed to conclude, in accordance with the inconsistency of the HPA data, that prolactin, but not the variables related to the HPA axis, is probably related to differences in active avoidance [143]. Even if RLA are characterized by a greater HPA reactivity, the possible influence of behavioral traits other than anxiety on the HPA axis should not be disregarded.

After inbreeding (RHA-I, RLA-I), we have reported normal resting levels of ACTH and corticosterone, but increased response of the two hormones to a novel environment [144]. Enhanced PVN CRH gene expression, but unaltered VP expression in PVNp and PVNm, was also observed in RLA-I versus RHA-I. Quite interestingly, enhanced CRH expression in the RLA-I rats was found in a brain area, the dorsolateral division of the bed nucleus of stria terminalis (BST). As the BST has been repeatedly implicated in the control of anxiety [13], our data suggest that extra-PVN changes in CRH gene expression may participate in some of the behavioral differences between the two strains.

Syracuse Low and Syracuse High avoidance (SLA, SHA) rats, have been also selectively bred on the basis of their behaviour in an active avoidance task (see [145]). Again, SLA and SHA rats appear to differ in emotionality. Thus, SLA rats defecate more in an open-field and show faster learning of a passive avoidance task and more fear conditioned suppression of appetitive instrumental behaviour than SHA, but no differences were observed in sensitivity to shock or activity. Unfortunately, it is not known whether they differ in anxiety as evaluated by the EPM. In accordance with their greater emotionality, SLA rats show a greater glucose response to an open-field [146]. However, SLA rats are characterized by modestly lower corticosterone response to ether stress, but much lower adrenal corticosterone content, as compared with SHA [147]. Similar results were observed after exogenous CRH administration [148]. Quite surprisingly, reduced adrenal corticosterone levels occur despite greater relative adrenal weight and greater size of adrenal cortex in SLA rats [148, 149]. The most likely explanation is that RLA showed a defective adrenocortical responsiveness to ACTH that tended to be compensated by increased adrenal mass. Unfortunately, ACTH levels were not measured in any experiment.

In conclusion, the comparison of the neuroendocrine characteristics of RLA-RHA and SLA-SHA is limited by the lack of information regarding the last pair of lines. Nevertheless, the available information does not reveal a homogenous pattern. Accordingly, in mice, the best performed studied compared several inbred strains of mice in several test for anxiety (EPM, ASR and hyponeophagia) and in basal and stress levels of corticosterone [150]. Whereas a good correlation among the strains was observed with the three tests of anxiety, no correlation was found between anxiety-like behaviour and corticosterone. These data support conclusions in rats.

4. General conclusions

The overall conclusion of the present review is that the physiological response does not reflect concomitant changes in objective anxiety as evaluated by classical tests in laboratory animals or self-reported measures in humans. There are several reasons that can explain such dissociation and the sometimes controversial results. First, the uncertainty about the underlying psychological or behavioral traits of interest and the way we can evaluate them.

Second, the use of animal lines differing in more than one trait, making difficult to separate the contribution of anxiety from that of other traits. Third, the different dynamics of the behavioral processes and the physiological variables measured. Four, the possibility that others, still not characterized, biological parameters may be more appropriate as biological correlates of anxiety. Finally, there are uncertainties about the relationship between subjective reports of anxiety and the biological response to aversive stimuli.

In laboratory animals, the classical approach has been the selection of the animals in function of particular criterium or test, assuming that this identifies the particular trait of interest, anxiety for the present discussion. However, it is unrealistic to assume that the selection of animals on the basis of one single test can really identify one particular trait. In addition, the experimental evidence strongly indicates that these animals also differ in other different traits, making it difficult to isolate anxiety for other traits. For instance, HAB-LAB rats not only differ in anxiety but also in depression-like behavior [124]. Similarly RLA and RHA rats also differ in impulsivity [137].

The most widely used physiological responses are those related to the SMA and the HPA axis, in addition to other hormones such as prolactin. The different indices greatly differ in terms of the time needed to reflect changes in the environment. Cardiovascular changes (i.e. HR, blood pressure) can rapidly change in one minute, plasma levels of adrenaline and noradrenaline is also very fast and their half-life is very short, thus resulting in the possibility of marked changes in periods of 5 minutes. Plasma levels of anterior pituitary hormones are released very fast (a few minutes), but half-life is longer than that of catecholamines (between 5 and 30 minutes or more, depending on the particular hormone). Finally, changes in plasma or salivary cortisol are relatively slow, with maximum no more than 15-30 minutes after the initial exposure to the situation. Thus, the dynamics of the response is important when considering the influence of cognitive processes in the regulation of the emotional response to the situation.

Although more elaborated endocrinological studies may help to elucidate some controversial results, it is important to look at other physiological variables. For instance, a recent study observed lower plasma levels of nesfatin-1, a recently characterized satiety molecule, in GAD patients [151]. Immunological markers are currently studied regarding stress and personality factors. In one interesting paper in a large population of men and women, anxiety positively correlated to levels of certain inflammatory markers (C-Reactive Protein, interleukin-6, Tumor Necrosis Factor-α and fibrinogen) [152]. Characterization of putative inflammatory markers of anxiety requires further studies.

In humans, psychological traits are complex constructs that involve top-down cognitive processes. In contrast, physiological response to aversive situations is likely to be reflexive in nature at least initially. It is possible that both processes are relatively independent. Rapid attention and responding to putatively threatening stimuli is a characteristic of several anxiety disorders and healthy people with high neuroticism or trait-anxiety [153]. In a very interesting study, preconscious and conscious attention biases to emotional stimuli were evaluated in subjects exposed 4 and 8 months later to a laboratory stressor or to examination, respectively [154]. Preconscious negative bias processing was a better predictor of cortisol response than self-reported neuroticism, trait-anxiety or extraversion.

Another additional problem when addressing human data is the limitation of the information we can obtain from typical laboratory stressors. First, emotional processing of stressors may be complex and dependent on the particular nature of the situation. Anxiety disorders may be associated to a differential processing of certain categories of stressors but not all stressors and therefore information obtain from exposure to standard stressors may be limited and different depending on the particular type of anxiety disorder. Second, laboratory stressors tend to be of lower intensity that some real-life stressors and it is unclear whether or not we can extrapolate the results from one type to the other.

Even if we can identify physiological variables related to pathological anxiety, an important concern is whether these variables are the consequence of the pathology or a predisposing factor. In the last year particular attention has been paid to this problem, but it is still an important drawback when analyzing published data.

Acknowledgements

This work was supported by grants from Ministerio de Economía y Competitividad (SAF2008-01175 and SAF2011-28313), Instituto de Salud Carlos III (RD06/0001/0015, Redes Temáticas de Investigación Cooperativa en Salud, Ministerio de Sanidad y Consumo), Plan Nacional sobre Drogas and Generalitat de Catalunya (SGR2009-16).

Author details

Antonio Armario[1*] and Roser Nadal[2]

*Address all correspondence to: Antonio.armario@uab.es

1 Institute of Neurosciencies and Animal Physiology Unit (Department of Cellular Biology, Physiology and Immunology, School of Biosciences), Universitat Autònoma de Barcelona, Barcelona, Spain

2 Institute of Neurosciencies and Psychobiology Unit (Department of Psychobiology and Methodology of Health Sciences, School of Psychology), Universitat Autònoma de Barcelona, Barcelona, Spain

References

[1] Costa PT, McCrae RR. NEO PI-R. Professional manual. Odessa, FL: Psychological Assessment Resources, Inc.; 1992.

[2] De Pauw SS, Mervielde I. Temperament, personality and developmental psychopathology: a review based on the conceptual dimensions underlying childhood traits. Child Psychiatry Hum Dev. 2010;41(3):313-29.

[3] Engelhard IM, van den Hout MA, Lommen MJJ. Individuals high in neuroticism are not more reactive to adverse events. Personality and Individual Differences 2009;47:697-700.

[4] Ramos A, Mormede P. Stress and emotionality: a multidimensional and genetic approach. Neurosci Biobehav Rev. 1998;22(1):33-57.

[5] Spielberger CD, Gorsuch RL, Lushene R, Vagg PR, Jacobs GA. Manual for the state-trait anxiety inventory. Palo Alto, CA: Conulting Psychology Press; 1983.

[6] Belzung C, Griebel G. Measuring normal and pathological anxiety-like behaviour in mice: a review. Behav Brain Res. 2001;125(1-2):141-9.

[7] Mineur YS, Belzung C, Crusio WE. Effects of unpredictable chronic mild stress on anxiety and depression-like behavior in mice. Behav Brain Res. 2006;175(1):43-50.

[8] Aguilar R, Gil L, Flint J, Gray JA, Dawson GR, Driscoll P, et al. Learned fear, emotional reactivity and fear of heights: a factor analytic map from a large F(2) intercross of Roman rat strains. Brain Res Bull. 2002;57(1):17-26.

[9] Kanari K, Kikusui T, Takeuchi Y, Mori Y. Multidimensional structure of anxiety-related behavior in early-weaned rats. Behav Brain Res. 2005;156(1):45-52.

[10] Griebel G, Simiand J, Serradeil-Le Gal C, Wagnon J, Pascal M, Scatton B, et al. Anxiolytic- and antidepressant-like effects of the non-peptide vasopressin V1b receptor antagonist, SSR149415, suggest an innovative approach for the treatment of stress-related disorders. Proc Natl Acad Sci U S A 2002;99(9):6370-5.

[11] Weisstaub NV, Zhou M, Lira A, Lambe E, Gonzalez-Maeso J, Hornung JP, et al. Cortical 5-HT2A receptor signaling modulates anxiety-like behaviors in mice. Science 2006;313(5786):536-40.

[12] Grillon C. Models and mechanisms of anxiety: evidence from startle studies. Psychopharmacology 2008;199(3):421-37.

[13] Davis M, Walker DL, Miles L, Grillon C. Phasic vs sustained fear in rats and humans: role of the extended amygdala in fear vs anxiety. Neuropsychopharmacology 2010;35(1):105-35.

[14] Pellow S, Chopin P, File SE, Briley M. Validation of open:closed arm entries in an elevated plus-maze as a measure of anxiety in the rat. J Neurosci Methods 1985;14(3): 149-67.

[15] Pellow S, File SE. Anxiolytic and anxiogenic drug effects on exploratory activity in an elevated plus-maze: a novel test of anxiety in the rat. Pharmacol Biochem Behav. 1986;24(3):525-9.

[16] Belzung C, Le Pape G. Comparison of different behavioral test situations used in psychopharmacology for measurement of anxiety. Physiol Behav. 1994;56(3):623-8.

[17] Hascoet M, Bourin M, Nic Dhonnchadha BA. The mouse light-dark paradigm: a review. Prog Neuropsychopharmacol Biol Psychiatry 2001;25(1):141-66.

[18] Fernandez-Teruel A, Escorihuela RM, Nunez JF, Zapata A, Boix F, Salazar W, et al. The early acquisition of two-way (shuttle-box) avoidance as an anxiety-mediated behavior: psychopharmacological validation. Brain Res Bull. 1991;26(1):173-6.

[19] Koolhaas JM, Korte SM, De Boer SF, Van Der Vegt BJ, Van Reenen CG, Hopster H, et al. Coping styles in animals: current status in behavior and stress-physiology. Neurosci Biobehav Rev. 1999;23(7):925-35.

[20] Steimer T, la Fleur S, Schulz PE. Neuroendocrine correlates of emotional reactivity and coping in male rats from the Roman high (RHA/Verh)- and low (RLA/Verh)-avoidance lines. Behav Genet. 1997;27(6):503-12.

[21] Mormede P, Foury A, Barat P, Corcuff JB, Terenina E, Marissal-Arvy N, et al. Molecular genetics of hypothalamic-pituitary-adrenal axis activity and function. Ann N Y Acad Sci. 2011;1220:127-36.

[22] Johnson EO, Kamilaris TC, Chrousos GP, Gold PW. Mechanisms of stress: a dynamic overview of hormonal and behavioral homeostasis. Neurosci Biobehav Rev. 1992;16(2):115-30.

[23] Valentino RJ, Miselis RR, Pavcovich LA. Pontine regulation of pelvic viscera: pharmacological target for pelvic visceral dysfunctions. Trends Pharmacol Sci. 1999 Jun; 20(6):253-60.

[24] Rogers RC, Hermann GE, Travagli RA. Stress and the colon: central-vagal or direct peripheral effect of CRF? Am J Physiol Regul Integr Comp Physiol. 2006;290(6):R1535-6.

[25] Tsukamoto K, Nakade Y, Mantyh C, Ludwig K, Pappas TN, Takahashi T. Peripherally administered CRF stimulates colonic motility via central CRF receptors and vagal pathways in conscious rats. Am J Physiol Regul Integr Comp Physiol. 2006;290(6):R1537-41.

[26] Morrison SF. Differential control of sympathetic outflow. Am J Physiol Regul Integr Comp Physiol. 2001;281(3):R683-98.

[27] Saper CB. The central autonomic nervous system: conscious visceral perception and autonomic pattern generation. Annu Rev Neurosci. 2002;25:433-69.

[28] Kreibig SD. Autonomic nervous system activity in emotion: a review. Biol Psychol. 2010;84(3):394-421.

[29] Armario A, Daviu N, Munoz-Abellan C, Rabasa C, Fuentes S, Belda X, et al. What can we know from pituitary-adrenal hormones about the nature and consequences of exposure to emotional stressors? Cell Mol Neurobiol. 2012;32(5):749-58.

[30] Armario A. The hypothalamic-pituitary-adrenal axis: what can it tell us about stressors? CNS Neurol Disord Drug Targets 2006;5(5):485-501.

[31] Marquez C, Nadal R, Armario A. The hypothalamic-pituitary-adrenal and glucose responses to daily repeated immobilisation stress in rats: individual differences. Neuroscience. 2004;123(3):601-12.

[32] de Kloet ER, Reul JM, Sutanto W. Corticosteroids and the brain. J Steroid Biochem Mol Biol. 1990;37(3):387-94.

[33] Makara GB, Haller J. Non-genomic effects of glucocorticoids in the neural system. Evidence, mechanisms and implications. Prog Neurobiol. 2001;65(4):367-90.

[34] Keller-Wood ME, Dallman MF. Corticosteroid inhibition of ACTH secretion. Endocr Rev. 1984;5(1):1-24.

[35] Pariante CM. The role of multi-drug resistance p-glycoprotein in glucocorticoid function: studies in animals and relevance in humans. Eur J Pharmacol. 2008;583(2-3): 263-71.

[36] Young EA, Abelson J, Lightman SL. Cortisol pulsatility and its role in stress regulation and health. Front Neuroendocrinol. 2004;25(2):69-76.

[37] Ulrich-Lai YM, Arnhold MM, Engeland WC. Adrenal splanchnic innervation contributes to the diurnal rhythm of plasma corticosterone in rats by modulating adrenal sensitivity to ACTH. Am J Physiol Regul Integr Comp Physiol. 2006;290(4):R1128-35.

[38] Fries E, Dettenborn L, Kirschbaum C. The cortisol awakening response (CAR): facts and future directions. Int J Psychophysiol. 2009;72(1):67-73.

[39] Clow A, Hucklebridge F, Stalder T, Evans P, Thorn L. The cortisol awakening response: more than a measure of HPA axis function. Neurosci Biobehav Rev. 2010;35(1):97-103.

[40] Marti O, Armario A. Anterior pituitary response to stress: time-related changes and adaptation. Int J Dev Neurosci. 1998;16(3-4):241-60.

[41] Sternberg EM, Hill JM, Chrousos GP, Kamilaris T, Listwak SJ, Gold PW, et al. Inflammatory mediator-induced hypothalamic-pituitary-adrenal axis activation is defective in streptococcal cell wall arthritis-susceptible Lewis rats. Proc Natl Acad Sci U S A 1989;86(7):2374-8.

[42] Armario A, Gavalda A, Marti J. Comparison of the behavioural and endocrine response to forced swimming stress in five inbred strains of rats. Psychoneuroendocrinology 1995;20(8):879-90.

[43] Grattan DR, Kokay IC. Prolactin: a pleiotropic neuroendocrine hormone. J Neuroendocrinol. 2008;20(6):752-63.

[44] Torner L, Toschi N, Pohlinger A, Landgraf R, Neumann ID. Anxiolytic and anti-stress effects of brain prolactin: improved efficacy of antisense targeting of the prolactin receptor by molecular modeling. J Neurosci. 2001;21(9):3207-14.

[45] Li HY, Ericsson A, Sawchenko PE. Distinct mechanisms underlie activation of hypothalamic neurosecretory neurons and their medullary catecholaminergic afferents in categorically different stress paradigms. Proc Natl Acad Sci U S A 1996;93(6):2359-64.

[46] Ulrich-Lai YM, Herman JP. Neural regulation of endocrine and autonomic stress responses. Nat Rev Neurosci. 2009;10(6):397-409.

[47] Pacak K, Palkovits M. Stressor specificity of central neuroendocrine responses: implications for stress-related disorders. Endocr Rev. 2001;22(4):502-48.

[48] Armario A, Lopez-Calderon A, Jolin T, Castellanos JM. Sensitivity of anterior pituitary hormones to graded levels of psychological stress. Life Sci. 1986;39(5):471-5.

[49] Noel GL, Dimond RC, Earll JM, Frantz AG. Prolactin, thyrotropin, and growth hormone release during stress associated with parachute jumping. Aviat Space Environ Med. 1976;47(5):534-7.

[50] Schedlowski M, Wiechert D, Wagner TO, Tewes U. Acute psychological stress increases plasma levels of cortisol, prolactin and TSH. Life Sci. 1992;50(17):1201-5.

[51] Chatterton RT, Jr., Vogelsong KM, Lu YC, Hudgens GA. Hormonal responses to psychological stress in men preparing for skydiving. J Clin Endocrinol Metab. 1997;82(8): 2503-9.

[52] Marquez C, Nadal R, Armario A. Responsiveness of the hypothalamic-pituitary-adrenal axis to different novel environments is a consistent individual trait in adult male outbred rats. Psychoneuroendocrinology 2005;30(2):179-87.

[53] Marquez C, Nadal R, Armario A. Influence of reactivity to novelty and anxiety on hypothalamic-pituitary-adrenal and prolactin responses to two different novel environments in adult male rats. Behav Brain Res. 2006;168(1):13-22.

[54] Callister R, Suwarno NO, Seals DR. Sympathetic activity is influenced by task difficulty and stress perception during mental challenge in humans. J Physiol. 1992;454:373-87.

[55] Armario A, Marti O, Molina T, de Pablo J, Valdes M. Acute stress markers in humans: response of plasma glucose, cortisol and prolactin to two examinations differing in the anxiety they provoke. Psychoneuroendocrinology 1996;21(1):17-24.

[56] Morgan CA, 3rd, Wang S, Mason J, Southwick SM, Fox P, Hazlett G, et al. Hormone profiles in humans experiencing military survival training. Biol Psychiatry 2000;47(10):891-901.

[57] Foley P, Kirschbaum C. Human hypothalamus-pituitary-adrenal axis responses to acute psychosocial stress in laboratory settings. Neurosci Biobehav Rev. 2010;35(1): 91-6.

[58] Schommer NC, Hellhammer DH, Kirschbaum C. Dissociation between reactivity of the hypothalamus-pituitary-adrenal axis and the sympathetic-adrenal-medullary system to repeated psychosocial stress. Psychosom Med. 2003;65(3):450-60.

[59] Lerner JS, Gonzalez RM, Dahl RE, Hariri AR, Taylor SE. Facial expressions of emotion reveal neuroendocrine and cardiovascular stress responses. Biol Psychiatry 2005;58(9):743-50.

[60] Dickerson SS, Kemeny ME. Acute stressors and cortisol responses: a theoretical integration and synthesis of laboratory research. Psychol Bull. 2004;130(3):355-91.

[61] Brooks JE, Herbert M, Walder CP, Selby C, Jeffcoate WJ. Prolactin and stress: some endocrine correlates of pre-operative anxiety. Clin Endocrinol. 1986;24(6):653-6.

[62] Cohen S, Hamrick N, Rodriguez MS, Feldman PJ, Rabin BS, Manuck SB. The stability of and intercorrelations among cardiovascular, immune, endocrine, and psychological reactivity. Ann Behav Med. 2000;22(3):171-9.

[63] Pottier P, Hardouin JB, Dejoie T, Bonnaud A, Le Loupp AG, Planchon B, et al. Stress responses in medical students in ambulatory and in-hospital patient consultations. Med Educ. 2011;45(7):678-87.

[64] Hellhammer J, Schubert M. The physiological response to Trier Social Stress Test relates to subjective measures of stress during but not before or after the test. Psychoneuroendocrinology 2012;37(1):119-24.

[65] Noto Y, Sato T, Kudo M, Kurata K, Hirota K. The relationship between salivary biomarkers and state-trait anxiety inventory score under mental arithmetic stress: a pilot study. Anesth Analg. 2005;101(6):1873-6.

[66] Arora S, Tierney T, Sevdalis N, Aggarwal R, Nestel D, Woloshynowych M, et al. The Imperial Stress Assessment Tool (ISAT): a feasible, reliable and valid approach to measuring stress in the operating room. World J Surg. 2010;34(8):1756-63.

[67] Detling N, Smith A, Nishimura R, Keller S, Martinez M, Young W, et al. Psychophysiologic responses of invasive cardiologists in an academic catheterization laboratory. Am Heart J. 2006;151(2):522-8.

[68] van Eck MM, Nicolson NA, Berkhof H, Sulon J. Individual differences in cortisol responses to a laboratory speech task and their relationship to responses to stressful daily events. Biol Psychol. 1996;43(1):69-84.

[69] Wirtz PH, Elsenbruch S, Emini L, Rudisuli K, Groessbauer S, Ehlert U. Perfectionism and the cortisol response to psychosocial stress in men. Psychosom Med. 2007;69(3): 249-55.

[70] Buske-Kirschbaum A, Ebrecht M, Kern S, Gierens A, Hellhammer DH. Personality characteristics in chronic and non-chronic allergic conditions. Brain Behav Immun. 2008;22(5):762-8.

[71] Maruyama Y, Kawano A, Okamoto S, Ando T, Ishitobi Y, Tanaka Y, et al. Differences in salivary alpha-amylase and cortisol responsiveness following exposure to electrical stimulation versus the Trier Social Stress tests. PLoS One 2012;7(7):e39375.

[72] Hubert W, de Jong-Meyer R. Saliva cortisol responses to unpleasant film stimuli differ between high and low trait anxious subjects. Neuropsychobiology 1992;25(2): 115-20.

[73] Jezova D, Makatsori A, Duncko R, Moncek F, Jakubek M. High trait anxiety in healthy subjects is associated with low neuroendocrine activity during psychosocial stress. Prog Neuropsychopharmacol Biol Psychiatry 2004;28(8):1331-6.

[74] Duncko R, Makatsori A, Fickova E, Selko D, Jezova D. Altered coordination of the neuroendocrine response during psychosocial stress in subjects with high trait anxiety. Prog Neuropsychopharmacol Biol Psychiatry 2006;30(6):1058-66.

[75] de Rooij SR, Schene AH, Phillips DI, Roseboom TJ. Depression and anxiety: Associations with biological and perceived stress reactivity to a psychological stress protocol in a middle-aged population. Psychoneuroendocrinology 2010;35(6):866-77.

[76] Katsuura S, Kamezaki Y, Yamagishi N, Kuwano Y, Nishida K, Masuda K, et al. Circulating vascular endothelial growth factor is independently and negatively associated with trait anxiety and depressive mood in healthy Japanese university students. Int J Psychophysiol. 2011;81(1):38-43.

[77] Tyrka AR, Wier LM, Price LH, Rikhye K, Ross NS, Anderson GM, et al. Cortisol and ACTH responses to the Dex/CRH test: influence of temperament. Horm Behav. 2008;53(4):518-25.

[78] Taylor MK, Reis JP, Sausen KP, Padilla GA, Markham AE, Potterat EG, et al. Trait anxiety and salivary cortisol during free living and military stress. Aviat Space Environ Med. 2008;79(2):129-35.

[79] Van den Bergh BR, Van Calster B, Pinna Puissant S, Van Huffel S. Self-reported symptoms of depressed mood, trait anxiety and aggressive behavior in post-pubertal adolescents: Associations with diurnal cortisol profiles. Horm Behav. 2008;54(2): 253-7.

[80] Takai N, Yamaguchi M, Aragaki T, Eto K, Uchihashi K, Nishikawa Y. Effect of psychological stress on the salivary cortisol and amylase levels in healthy young adults. Arch Oral Biol. 2004;49(12):963-8.

[81] Allwood MA, Handwerger K, Kivlighan KT, Granger DA, Stroud LR. Direct and moderating links of salivary alpha-amylase and cortisol stress-reactivity to youth behavioral and emotional adjustment. Biol Psychol. 2011;88(1):57-64.

[82] Diagnostic and Statistical Manual of Mental Disorders, Fourth Edition, Text Revision. Washington, D.C.: American Psychiatric Association; 2000.

[83] Curtis GC, Glitz DA. Neuroendocrine findings in anxiety disorders. Endocrinology and Metabolism Clinics of North America; 1988. p. 131-48.

[84] Tollefson GD. Buspirone: effects on prolactin and growth hormone as a function of drug level in generalized anxiety. J Clin Psychopharmacol. 1989;9(5):387.

[85] Fossey MD, Lydiard RB, Ballenger JC, Laraia MT, Bissette G, Nemeroff CB. Cerebrospinal fluid corticotropin-releasing factor concentrations in patients with anxiety disorders and normal comparison subjects. Biol Psychiatry. 1996;39(8):703-7.

[86] Mantella RC, Butters MA, Amico JA, Mazumdar S, Rollman BL, Begley AE, et al. Salivary cortisol is associated with diagnosis and severity of late-life generalized anxiety disorder. Psychoneuroendocrinology 2008;33(6):773-81.

[87] Vreeburg SA, Zitman FG, van Pelt J, Derijk RH, Verhagen JC, van Dyck R, et al. Salivary cortisol levels in persons with and without different anxiety disorders. Psychosom Med. 2010;72(4):340-7.

[88] Hek K, Direk N, Newson RS, Hofman A, Hoogendijk WJ, Mulder CL, et al. Anxiety disorders and salivary cortisol levels in older adults: a population-based study. Psychoneuroendocrinology 2012 Epub ahead of print.

[89] van Veen JF, van Vliet IM, Derijk RH, van Pelt J, Mertens B, Zitman FG. Elevated alpha-amylase but not cortisol in generalized social anxiety disorder. Psychoneuroendocrinology 2008;33(10):1313-21.

[90] Steudte S, Stalder T, Dettenborn L, Klumbies E, Foley P, Beesdo-Baum K, et al. Decreased hair cortisol concentrations in generalised anxiety disorder. Psychiatry Res. 2011;186(2-3):310-4.

[91] Abelson JL, Curtis GC. Hypothalamic-pituitary-adrenal axis activity in panic disorder. 24-hour secretion of corticotropin and cortisol. Arch Gen Psychiatry 1996;53(4): 323-31.

[92] Gerra G, Zaimovic A, Zambelli U, Timpano M, Reali N, Bernasconi S, et al. Neuroendocrine responses to psychological stress in adolescents with anxiety disorder. Neuropsychobiology 2000;42(2):82-92.

[93] Nesse RM, Curtis GC, Brown GM, Rubin RT. Anxiety induced by flooding therapy for phobias does not elicit prolactin secretory response. Psychosom Med. 1980;42(1): 25-31.

[94] Nesse RM, Curtis GC, Thyer BA, McCann DS, Huber-Smith MJ, Knopf RF. Endocrine and cardiovascular responses during phobic anxiety. Psychosom Med. 1985;47(4): 320-32.

[95] Van Duinen MA, Schruers KR, Griez EJ. Desynchrony of fear in phobic exposure. J Psychopharmacol. 2010;24(5):695-9.

[96] Alpers GW, Abelson JL, Wilhelm FH, Roth WT. Salivary cortisol response during exposure treatment in driving phobics. Psychosom Med. 2003;65(4):679-87.

[97] Martel FL, Hayward C, Lyons DM, Sanborn K, Varady S, Schatzberg AF.Salivary cortisol levels in socially phobic adolescent girls. Depress Anxiety 1999;10(1):25-7.

[98] van West D, Claes S, Sulon J, Deboutte D. Hypothalamic-pituitary-adrenal reactivity in prepubertal children with social phobia. J Affect Disord. 2008;111(2-3):281-90.

[99] Kramer M, Seefeldt WL, Heinrichs N, Tuschen-Caffier B, Schmitz J, Wolf OT, et al. Subjective, autonomic, and endocrine reactivity during social stress in children with social phobia. J Abnorm Child Psychol. 2012;40(1):95-104.

[100] Roelofs K, Van Peer J, Berretty E, Jong P, Spinhoven P, Elzinga BM. Hypothalamus-pituitary-adrenal hyperresponsiveness is associated with increased social avoidance behavior in social phobia. Biol Psychiatry 2009;65(4):336-43.

[101] Cameron OG, Lee MA, Curtis GC, McCann DS. Endocrine and physiological changes during "spontaneous" panic attacks. Psychoneuroendocrinology 1987;12(5):321-31.

[102] Woods SW, Charney DS, McPherson CA, Gradman AH, Heninger GR. Situational panic attacks. Behavioral, physiologic, and biochemical characterization. Arch Gen Psychiatry 1987;44(4):365-75.

[103] Targum SD, Marshall LE. Fenfluramine provocation of anxiety in patients with panic disorder. Psychiatry Res. 1989;28(3):295-306.

[104] Liebowitz MR, Gorman JM, Fyer AJ, Levitt M, Dillon D, Levy G, et al. Lactate provocation of panic attacks. II. Biochemical and physiological findings. Arch Gen Psychiatry 1985;42(7):709-19.

[105] Carr DB, Sheehan DV, Surman OS, Coleman JH, Greenblatt DJ, Heninger GR, et al. Neuroendocrine correlates of lactate-induced anxiety and their response to chronic alprazolam therapy. Am J Psychiatry 1986;143(4):483-94.

[106] Woods SW, Charney DS, Goodman WK, Heninger GR. Carbon dioxide-induced anxiety. Behavioral, physiologic, and biochemical effects of carbon dioxide in patients with panic disorders and healthy subjects. Arch Gen Psychiatry 1988;45(1): 43-52.

[107] Hollander E, Liebowitz MR, Cohen B, Gorman JM, Fyer AJ, Papp LA, et al. Prolactin and sodium lactate-induced panic. Psychiatry Res. 1989;28(2):181-91.

[108] Koszycki D, Zacharko RM, Le Melledo JM, Bradwejn J. Behavioral, cardiovascular, and neuroendocrine profiles following CCK-4 challenge in healthy volunteers: a comparison of panickers and nonpanickers. Depress Anxiety 1998;8(1):1-7.

[109] Abelson JL, Liberzon I, Young EA, Khan S. Cognitive modulation of the endocrine stress response to a pharmacological challenge in normal and panic disorder subjects. Arch Gen Psychiatry 2005;62(6):668-75.

[110] Gutman DA, Coplan J, Papp L, Martinez J, Gorman J. Doxapram-induced panic attacks and cortisol elevation. Psychiatry Res. 2005;133(2-3):253-61.

[111] Van Veen JF, Van der Wee NJ, Fiselier J, Van Vliet IM, Westenberg HG. Behavioural effects of rapid intravenous administration of meta-chlorophenylpiperazine (m-CPP) in patients with generalized social anxiety disorder, panic disorder and healthy controls. Eur Neuropsychopharmacol. 2007;17(10):637-42.

[112] Leyton M, Belanger C, Martial J, Beaulieu S, Corin E, Pecknold J, et al. Cardiovascular, neuroendocrine, and monoaminergic responses to psychological stressors: possible differences between remitted panic disorder patients and healthy controls. Biol Psychiatry 1996;40(5):353-60.

[113] Parente AC, Garcia-Leal C, Del-Ben CM, Guimaraes FS, Graeff FG. Subjective and neurovegetative changes in healthy volunteers and panic patients performing simulated public speaking. Eur Neuropsychopharmacol. 2005;15(6):663-71.

[114] Garcia-Leal C, Parente AC, Del-Ben CM, Guimaraes FS, Moreira AC, Elias LL, et al. Anxiety and salivary cortisol in symptomatic and nonsymptomatic panic patients and healthy volunteers performing simulated public speaking. Psychiatry Res. 2005;133(2-3):239-52.

[115] Petrowski K, Herold U, Joraschky P, Wittchen HU, Kirschbaum C. A striking pattern of cortisol non-responsiveness to psychosocial stress in patients with panic disorder with concurrent normal cortisol awakening responses. Psychoneuroendocrinology 2010;35(3):414-21.

[116] Tanaka Y, Ishitobi Y, Maruyama Y, Kawano A, Ando T, Imanaga J, et al. Salivary alpha-amylase and cortisol responsiveness following electrical stimulation stress in panic disorder patients. Neurosci Res. 2012;73(1):80-4.

[117] Blizard DA, Adams N. The Maudsley Reactive and Nonreactive strains: a new perspective. Behav Genet. 2002;32(5):277-99.

[118] Beardslee SL, Papadakis E, Altman HJ, Harrington GM, Commissaris RL. Defensive burying behavior in maudsley reactive (MR/Har) and nonreactive (MNRA/Har) rats. Physiol Behav. 1989;45(2):449-51.

[119] Commissaris RL, Franklin L, Verbanac JS, Altman HJ. Maudsley reactive (MR/Har) and nonreactive (MNRA/Har) rats: performance in an operant conflict paradigm. Physiol Behav. 1992;52(5):873-8.

[120] Overstreet DH, Rezvani AH, Janowsky DS. Maudsley reactive and nonreactive rats differ only in some tasks reflecting emotionality. Physiol Behav. 1992;52(1):149-52.

[121] Paterson A, Whiting PJ, Gray JA, Flint J, Dawson GR. Lack of consistent behavioural effects of Maudsley reactive and non-reactive rats in a number of animal tests of anxiety and activity. Psychopharmacology 2001;154(4):336-42.

[122] Abel EL. Behavior and corticosteroid response of Maudsley reactive and nonreactive rats in the open field and forced swimming test. Physiol Behav. 1991;50(1):151-3.

[123] Kosti O, Raven PW, Renshaw D, Hinson JP. Intra-adrenal mechanisms in the response to chronic stress: investigation in a rat model of emotionality. J Endocrinol. 2006;189(2):211-8.

[124] Liebsch G, Montkowski A, Holsboer F, Landgraf R. Behavioural profiles of two Wistar rat lines selectively bred for high or low anxiety-related behaviour. Behav Brain Res. 1998;94(2):301-10.

[125] Henniger MS, Ohl F, Holter SM, Weissenbacher P, Toschi N, Lorscher P, et al. Unconditioned anxiety and social behaviour in two rat lines selectively bred for high and low anxiety-related behaviour. Behav Brain Res. 2000;111(1-2):153-63.

[126] Liebsch G, Linthorst AC, Neumann ID, Reul JM, Holsboer F, Landgraf R. Behavioral, physiological, and neuroendocrine stress responses and differential sensitivity to diazepam in two Wistar rat lines selectively bred for high- and low-anxiety-related behavior. Neuropsychopharmacology 1998;19(5):381-96.

[127] Porsolt RD, Le Pichon M, Jalfre M. Depression: a new animal model sensitive to antidepressant treatments. Nature 1977;266(5604):730-2.

[128] Marti J, Armario A. Effects of diazepam and desipramine in the forced swimming test: influence of previous experience with the situation. Eur J Pharmacol. 1993;236(2):295-9.

[129] Landgraf R, Wigger A, Holsboer F, Neumann ID. Hyper-reactive hypothalamo-pituitary-adrenocortical axis in rats bred for high anxiety-related behaviour. J Neuroendocrinol. 1999;11(6):405-7.

[130] Frank E, Salchner P, Aldag JM, Salome N, Singewald N, Landgraf R, et al. Genetic predisposition to anxiety-related behavior determines coping style, neuroendocrine responses, and neuronal activation during social defeat. Behav Neurosci. 2006;120(1): 60-71.

[131] Keck ME, Wigger A, Welt T, Muller MB, Gesing A, Reul JM, et al. Vasopressin mediates the response of the combined dexamethasone/CRH test in hyper-anxious rats: implications for pathogenesis of affective disorders. Neuropsychopharmacology 2002;26(1):94-105.

[132] Bosch OJ, Kromer SA, Neumann ID. Prenatal stress: opposite effects on anxiety and hypothalamic expression of vasopressin and corticotropin-releasing hormone in rats selectively bred for high and low anxiety. Eur J Neurosci. 2006;23(2):541-51.

[133] Salome N, Viltart O, Lesage J, Landgraf R, Vieau D, Laborie C. Altered hypothalamo-pituitary-adrenal and sympatho-adrenomedullary activities in rats bred for high anxiety: central and peripheral correlates. Psychoneuroendocrinology 2006;31(6): 724-35.

[134] Wigger A, Sanchez MM, Mathys KC, Ebner K, Frank E, Liu D, et al. Alterations in central neuropeptide expression, release, and receptor binding in rats bred for high anxiety: critical role of vasopressin. Neuropsychopharmacology 2004;29(1):1-14.

[135] Keck ME, Welt T, Post A, Muller MB, Toschi N, Wigger A, et al. Neuroendocrine and behavioral effects of repetitive transcranial magnetic stimulation in a psychopathological animal model are suggestive of antidepressant-like effects. Neuropsychopharmacology 2001;24(4):337-49.

[136] Salome N, Tasiemski A, Dutriez I, Wigger A, Landgraf R, Viltart O. Immune challenge induces differential corticosterone and interleukin-6 responsiveness in rats bred for extremes in anxiety-related behavior. Neuroscience 2008;151(4):1112-8.

[137] Steimer T, Driscoll P. Divergent stress responses and coping styles in psychogenetically selected Roman high-(RHA) and low-(RLA) avoidance rats: behavioural, neuroendocrine and developmental aspects. Stress 2003;6(2):87-100.

[138] Gentsch C, Lichtsteiner M, Driscoll P, Feer H. Differential hormonal and physiological responses to stress in Roman high- and low-avoidance rats. Physiol Behav. 1982;28(2):259-63.

[139] Castanon N, Dulluc J, le Moal M, Mormede P. Prolactin as a link between behavioral and immune differences between the Roman rat lines. Physiol Behav. 1992;51(6): 1235-41.

[140] Castanon N, Dulluc J, Le Moal M, Mormede P. Maturation of the behavioral and neuroendocrine differences between the Roman rat lines. Physiol Behav. 1994;55(4): 775-82.

[141] Walker CD, Rivest RW, Meaney MJ, Aubert ML. Differential activation of the pituitary-adrenocortical axis after stress in the rat: use of two genetically selected lines (Roman low- and high-avoidance rats) as a model. J Endocrinol. 1989;123(3):477-85.

[142] Aubry JM, Bartanusz V, Driscoll P, Schulz P, Steimer T, Kiss JZ. Corticotropin-releasing factor and vasopressin mRNA levels in roman high- and low-avoidance rats: response to open-field exposure. Neuroendocrinology. 1995;61(2):89-97.

[143] Castanon N, Perez-Diaz F, Mormede P. Genetic analysis of the relationships between behavioral and neuroendocrine traits in Roman High and Low Avoidance rat lines. Behav Genet. 1995;25(4):371-84.

[144] Carrasco J, Marquez C, Nadal R, Tobena A, Fernandez-Teruel A, Armario A. Characterization of central and peripheral components of the hypothalamus-pituitary-adrenal axis in the inbred Roman rat strains. Psychoneuroendocrinology 2008;33(4): 437-45.

[145] Brush FR. Selection for differences in avoidance learning: the Syracuse strains differ in anxiety, not learning ability. Behav Genet. 2003;33(6):677-96.

[146] Flaherty CF, Rowan GA. Rats (Rattus norvegicus) selectively bred to differ in avoidance behavior also differ in response to novelty stress, in glycemic conditioning, and in reward contrast. Behav Neural Biol. 1989;51(2):145-64.

[147] Brush FR, Isaacson MD, Pellegrino LJ, Rykaszewski IM, Shain CN. Characteristics of the pituitary-adrenal system in the Syracuse high- and low-avoidance strains of rats (Rattus norvegicus). Behav Genet. 1991;21(1):35-48.

[148] Gupta P, Brush FR. Differential behavioral and endocrinological effects of corticotropin-releasing hormone (CRH) in the Syracuse high- and low-avoidance rats. Horm Behav. 1998;34(3):262-7.

[149] Del Paine SN, Brush FR. Adrenal morphometry in unilateral and sham adrenalectomized Syracuse high and low avoidance rats. Physiol Behav. 1990;48(2):299-306.

[150] Trullas R, Skolnick P. Differences in fear motivated behaviors among inbred mouse strains. Psychopharmacology 1993;111(3):323-31.

[151] Gunay H, Tutuncu R, Aydin S, Dag E, Abasli D. Decreased plasma nesfatin-1 levels in patients with generalized anxiety disorder. Psychoneuroendocrinology 2012 Epub ahead of print.

[152] Pitsavos C, Panagiotakos DB, Papageorgiou C, Tsetsekou E, Soldatos C, Stefanadis C. Anxiety in relation to inflammation and coagulation markers, among healthy adults: the ATTICA study. Atherosclerosis 2006;185(2):320-6.

[153] MacLeod C, Mathews A. Cognitive bias modification approaches to anxiety. Annu Rev Clin Psychol. 2012;8:189-217.

[154] Fox E, Cahill S, Zougkou K. Preconscious processing biases predict emotional reactivity to stress. Biol Psychiatry 2010;67(4):371-7.

Chapter 4

Focusing on the Possible Role of the Cerebellum in Anxiety Disorders

Meghan D. Caulfield and Richard J. Servatius

Additional information is available at the end of the chapter

1. Introduction

The cerebellum is traditionally thought of as the neural structure responsible for motor control, voluntary movement, balance and associative learning. However, there is a growing awareness that the cerebellum plays a role in higher cognitive functions such as sensory processing [1,2], attention [3,4], verbal working memory [5-8] and emotion [9-11]. Converging evidence suggests that the cerebellum may play a role in anxiety disorders. With the greater appreciation that anxiety disorders are best conceptualized by diathesis models of risk, cerebellar activation may represent an endophenotype contributing to anxiety etiology.

This chapter will present the role of a normal functioning cerebellum and outline instances in which abnormal functioning underlies a variety of pathologies including anxiety disorders. We will begin by describing historically accepted roles of the cerebellum in motor control, timing, and learning and memory. We will then present research relating to less appreciated roles such as executive processing and emotional control to demonstrate less recognized cognitive and emotional capacities of the cerebellum.

Key to our theory is that individual differences in cerebellar activity underlie vulnerability to develop anxiety disorders. This argument will be presented by providing an overview of pre-existing vulnerabilities contributing to a diathesis approach of anxiety. We will discuss recent research in which individual differences in cerebellar modulated activities is present, such as during associative learning, avoidance or image processing tasks. Finally, a diathesis model which incorporates cerebellar activation into the etiology and expression of anxiety disorders will be presented with a discussion of its implications and future directions.

2. Historically accepted roles of the cerebellum

The cerebellum is a unique neural structure that accounts for approximately 10% of the total brain volume and contains nearly half of all the neurons of the brain [12,13]. The cerebellum is highly organized, with distinct inputs and outputs. It is made up of an outer region of gray matter (the cerebellar cortex), an inner region of white matter, and three pairs of deep nuclei responsible for cerebellar output; the dentate, the fastigial, and the interposed[13]. The cerebellum is made up of two hemispheres that are structural mirror images, each containing three deep nuclei. The two hemispheres are connected medially by the vermis. For specificity, the cerebellum is segregated into sections: Crus I, Crus II, and lobules I-X ([14].

Motor Functioning. The traditional view of the cerebellum is that of a motor comparator. Muscle movement, especially coordinated and smooth motions, are the product of a feedback loop involving the cerebellum and frontal cortex. Afferent connections via the cortico-pontine-cerebellar tract with the premotor and motor cortex carry a "copy" of motor demands to the cerebellum. The cerebellum then compares feedback from the muscle spindles, joints, and tendons via the cerebellar peduncles to modify motor behavior, maintain coordination and perform skilled movements [15-17].

The essential role of the cerebellum in motor behavior is especially evident following cerebellar insult. Unlike lesions of the motor cortex, a cerebellar lesion does not eliminate movement entirely. Instead, it disrupts initiation, coordination, and timing of movements. Movement deficits following cerebellar lesions can be very precise. Some lesions affect certain muscle groups, but not others, depending on the location, revealing a precise topography in the cerebellum. For example, deterioration of the anterior cerebellum affects the lower limbs, causing a wide staggering gait, while largely sparing arm and hand movements [18-21]. Cerebellar lesions often lead to a lack of coordination, affecting the ability to perform directed movements. Damage to the vestibulocerebellum, which receives input from the vestibular nuclei, affects gross movements, such as standing upright, to fine movements, such as maintaining fixation of gaze. Spinocerebellar lesions disrupt signals from the spinal cord and affect coordination interfering with movement regulation. The spinocerebellum uses a feed-forward process to make on-line updates to ensure accurate coordinated movements. Lesions of the cerebellum cause a variety of movement disorders such as overshooting or undershooting of targets (referred to as dysmetria), poor path correction caused by poorly coordinated joint motions (known as ataxia), tremors at the end of actions [13,18,22]. Finally, insult of the cerebrocerebellum, which has afferents from the cerebral cortex, impairs planned movements and sensory input, affecting reaction time. Individuals with lesions to the cerebrocerebellum report difficulty performing directed actions. Instead of a smooth integration of movements toward a target, their actions take place as a series of several movements strung together, known as decomposition of movement [18]. Altogether, the profound and specific outcomes of cerebellar insult indicate its critical role in coordinated motor behavior, enabling smooth and accurate performance of highly specific fine motor movements.

Timing. Given its role in motor behaviors outlined above, it is not surprising that the cerebellum is essential in motor timing, which produces timed movements by coordinating velocity, acceleration and deceleration [15,23-28]. A simple way of measuring motor timing is through repetitive finger tapping tasks. Participants are asked to tap in time with a pacing device (e.g., metronome). After synchronization, the training device is removed and the individual is asked to continue tapping at the same interval. Variability in timing can then be measured in the inter-tap intervals. This simple task elucidates the essential role of the cerebellum in motor timing. Healthy participants demonstrate a significant increase in cerebellar activity (in addition to other areas related to motor timing such as the supplementary motor area and basal ganglia) during timed finger tapping [28]. Patients with lateral cerebellar lesions demonstrate increased variability when performing rhythmic tapping with the affected (ipsilateral) finger, but not when tapping with the unaffected (contralateral) finger. Interestingly, those with medial cerebellar lesions did not show timing errors, but had a greater number of motor errors, supporting involvement of the cerebellum specifically in timing and not just in producing the behavioral motor output [23].

Timing is also essential in higher cognitive functions such as stimulus processing, expectations, language, and attention. Sensory timing is often measured by duration judgment tasks, which presents two stimuli of either the same or different duration. Here, participants are required to attend to a stimulus, maintain it in working memory, compare it to a second stimulus and make a judgment. Significant increases in cerebellar activity are present during timing tasks in healthy human participants [29,30]. Additionally, the use of repetitive transcranial magnetic stimulation (rTMS), which induces inhibition and causes a "temporary lesion" in the stimulated region, of the lateral cerebellum impaired short interval time perception in a similar task (400-600 ms) [31]. Comparable sensory timing deficits are seen in children with Ataxia Telangiectasia, a disease involving cortical degeneration affecting Purkinje and granular cell layers [32]. A similar deficit in duration judgment is seen in patients with cerebellar tumors [33]. Furthermore, the effect of cerebellar lesions on sensory timing is not specific to duration judgment tasks. Patients with cerebellar lesions display deficits in a variety of other tasks requiring sensory processing including interval discrimination [24,34], speed judgments [35,36] and verbal timing [37-41].

Eyeblink conditioning. Although the cerebellum has long been acknowledged as a motor integrator and modulator, associative learning was assumed to be accomplished by higher cortical regions. Over the latter quarter of the 20th century, Thompson and colleagues presented a body of work that the cerebellum is part of the intrinsic circuitry for eyeblink conditioning, a form of new motor learning [42-45]. The foundation of eyeblink conditioning is the simple reflex pathway; the unconditional stimulus (US) produces an unconditional response (UR). Introduction of a second stimulus (conditioned stimulus or CS) that is temporally paired with the US gives rise to a conditioned response (CR), which precedes or significantly modifies the UR. In delay conditioning, the CS precedes and coterminates with the US. Thompson recognized that the simplicity of eyeblink conditioning coupled with the ability to explicitly assess reactivity to the CS, to the US, or its combination under various conditions provided an excellent platform to understand the nature of the engram – the storage and location of a memory trace [42,46,47].

The intrinsic cerebellar circuitry demonstrates why damage to the cerebellar cortex, cerebellar nuclei, or major afferent pathways abolishes or impairs acquisition of the CR during eyeblink conditioning [48-53]. Using rats and rabbits, the neurobiology of eyeblink conditioning has been reduced to two pathways that converge in the cerebellum (For detailed reviews see [45,54]). The basic essential pathway is presented in Figure 1. Simplified, the CS pathway transmits auditory, visual, and somatosensory information via the pontine nuclei to the cerebellar cortex and interpositus nucleus via mossy fiber connections. The US pathway takes two routes from the trigeminal nucleus: a reflexive route that bypasses the cerebellum and a learning route that integrates the relationship between the CS and US. From there, climbing fibers synapse at the cerebellar cortex and interpositus nucleus. The CS and US pathways converge in the cerebellar cortex and anterior interpositus. It is here where the memory trace is stored by changes in the firing patterns of purkinje cells during the development of the CR [47,55-57]. The CR is produced by release of inhibition of the interpositus, which increases activity to the red nucleus, in turn causing the cranial motor nuclei to induce an eye blink response [58,59].

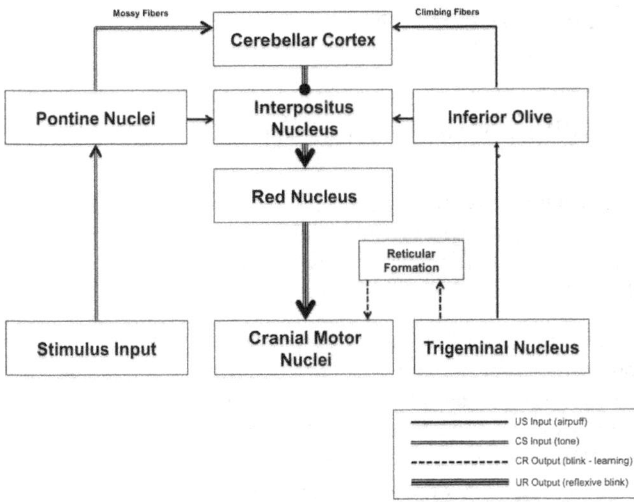

Figure 1. Intrinsic delay eyeblink conditioning pathway. Adapted from Christian & Thompson, 2003.

Another benefit of the eyeblink conditioning paradigm is that the same parameters can be used across animal species, in humans, and even in early infancy. Consistent with the animal literature, intact cerebellar structures are necessary for the acquisition of the CR in eyeblink conditioning in humans [48-50,60]. Furthermore, imaging studies indicate that activity in the cerebellum is significantly greater during eyeblink conditioning in humans [61-65].

Given the advanced understanding of neurosubstrates and its amenability for cross species comparisons, eyeblink conditioning has been a platform for understanding clinical abnormalities and cerebellar dysfunction. Therefore, a more detailed review will be presented for eyeblink conditioning, as well as a selection of clinical examples in which a cerebellar role is revealed by eyeblink conditioning.

Cerebellar abnormalities and eyeblink conditioning. The cerebellum is particularly affected by ethanol alcohol, with alcohol-related diseases causing serious damage to its development and cells. For example, impaired delay eyeblink conditioning has been observed in Korsakoff patients, recovered alcoholics, and children with Fetal Alcohol Syndrome [66-69]. However, not all disorders cause deficits in eyeblink conditioning. For example, individuals with autism acquire eyeblink conditioning faster than matched controls, although the form of the CR is altered [70,71]. Schizophrenia also alters cerebellar functioning, with facilitated eyeblink conditioning observed in schizophrenics compared to healthy controls [72]. Some interventions can also rescue or improve cerebellar functioning. For example, improved performance in eyeblink conditioning has been observed in mice following an antioxidant rich diet over a standard diet [73].

Regardless of etiology, cerebellar abnormalities affect eyeblink conditioning. The well-documented pathways, substrates, and lesion studies makes eyeblink conditioning a simple, yet sensitive tool to understand the cerebellar role in various neuropathologies.

3. Higher cognitive and emotional capacities

Recently, the cerebellum has garnered greater attention for its higher cognitive capabilities. Reviews such as those from Courchesne and colleagues [3,74], Schmahmann and colleagues [75,76] and others [77-79] establish the cognitive role of the cerebellum, which will be briefly summarized here.

Anatomy. In order to have a role in higher cognitive processing the cerebellum must maintain connections with neural structures known to influence cognition. As such, cerebellar efferents have been traced to both motor and non-motor areas of the frontal cortex [80-85]. Tract-tracing studies with primates indicate that cerebellar output to the dorsolateral prefrontal cortex (DLPFC) places it in a position to modulate higher cognitive processing. Transneuronal retrograde virus tracers injected into multiple areas of the DLPFC (Brodmann areas 9, 46 and 12) labeled neurons in the dentate nucleus, indicating that the dentate has output channels to prefrontal regions [84]. The DLPFC plays an important role in many aspects of executive functioning including organization [86,87], behavioral control [87] working memory [88,89], reasoning and decision making [90], reward and expectancy [91], and emotion and motivation [92]. Follow up studies were able to pinpoint lateral dentate projections to the prefrontal cortex (PFC), with separate dorsal dentate projections terminating in the motor and premotor regions, suggesting a topographic organization of the dentate nucleus with both motor and non-motor output to the cortex [93].

Functional connectivity. Cerebellar connectivity to non-motor cognitive areas in human imaging research reflects pathways implicated in primate studies. Functional connectivity MRI correlates signal fluctuations in one brain area with activity in another, implying a relationship between the two areas. Using this method, Allen et al. [94] found that activity in the dentate nucleus of the cerebellum correlated with changes in activity in non-motor regions such as the limbic system, parietal lobes, and prefrontal cortex. Connectivity between the cerebellum and anterior cingulate cortex, a region typically associated with error detection, anticipation, attention, and emotional responses, has also been reported in resting state paradigms [95]. Furthermore, there is evidence that the cerebellum contributes to the intrinsic connectivity networks, a series of brain structures that correspond to basic functions such as vision, audition, language, episodic memory, executive functioning, and salience detection [11]. Distinct contributions of the neocerebellum to the default mode network, the executive network, and the salience network substantiate the assertion that there is functional connectivity between the cerebellum and non-motor cognitive regions.

Clinical support for a cerebellar role in non-motor cognitive processes is established by the work of Schmahmann and colleagues. Schmahmann recognized that not all patients with cerebellar strokes present with motor deficits. By assessing motor impairments alongside stroke location, he found that individuals with posterior lobe lesions presented with minor if at any motor impairments. Instead, they suffered from behavioral changes affecting executive functioning, verbal fluency, working memory, abstract reasoning, spatial memory, personality, and language deficits; recently coined as *cerebellar cognitive affective syndrome* [96,97].

Loss of function in lesions is supported by activational studies in healthy humans. Using functional MRI, significant changes in cerebellar activity is present during tasks that are considered largely cognitive or to involve executive processing. Significant increases in cerebellar activity have been recorded during sensory timing [29,30], spatial attention [98-101], and verbal working memory tasks [5,6,102].

Anatomical and functional connectivity, specific activation during executive processing tasks, and impairments concomitant with lesions is convincing evidence that the cerebellum plays a critical role in higher cognitive processing.

Emotions. In addition to connections with prefrontal and frontal cortex, the cerebellum also has direct anatomical connections to the amygdala, the brain region typically associated with emotion and fear [103]. Functional support for this connectivity comes from imaging studies that demonstrate judging emotional intonation, feeling empathy, experiencing sadness, and viewing emotional pictures all correlate with increased activity in the cerebellum [9,76,104-106].

If the cerebellum has important connections to the limbic system, then it follows that stimulation of the cerebellum should result in changes of emotional behaviors. As such, electrical stimulation of the cerebellum in animals demonstrates that it is an important modulator of behaviors classically attributed to limbic functioning including grooming, eating, and sham rage [107-109]. Bernston et al. [107] reported that stimulating the cerebellum of cats induced grooming and eating behaviors, in addition to similar findings with rats [108,109]. The cerebellum, specifically the vermis, plays a role in fear and avoidant behaviors. For example, lesioning the vermis alters fear responses by decreasing freezing and increasing open field exploration [110]. On other other hand, stimulating the vermis induces fear responses, such as increased amplitude of the acoustic startle response [111], indicating cerebellar modulation of species-specific behaviors beyond coordination of muscle movements.

Reports from the clinical literature also support cerebellar modulation of emotion. Attempts to treat severe seizure disorders by stimulating the cerebellum provide unique case reports of observations about cerebellar functioning. Heath et al. [112] placed electrodes in the fastigial nucleus of an emotionally disturbed patient and observed increased activity in the region when the patient reported being angry or fearful. Descriptions of unpleasant sensations and the feeling of being scared were reported following stimulation of the dentate nucleus [113]. In a larger study of cerebellar stimulation as a treatment for chronic epilepsy, Cooper et al. [114] reported marked behavioral changes from sullen mood, dangerous, and aggressive behaviors to open, pleasant, responsive, and sociable affect in patients. More recently, descriptions of highly specific lesions to the cerebellar vermis includes personality changes, especially emotional effects such as flattening of affect [97,115]. Observations from these case studies suggest that the cerebellum may utilize its reciprocal connections with the prefrontal cortex and limbic system to modulate emotional processing.

Cerebellum and Anxiety Disorders

Anxiety. Anxiety is the most prevalent disorder in the United States with one quarter of the population estimated to develop an anxiety disorder at some time in their lives [116,117]. On the other hand, three quarters of the population does not suffer from clinical anxiety, raising the question what is it about an individual that makes them more likely to develop an anxiety disorder? Unfortunately, there is no single vulnerability increasing risk for anxiety. Instead, anxiety disorders are best represented by diathesis models, that is, preexisting conditions enhance risk such that individuals are vulnerable to environmental insults or challenges. A stress-diathesis model for anxiety disorders emphasizes changes in stress reactivity from the convergence of a variety of factors such as genetics, biology, sex, and prior experience [118]. Current research efforts heavily focus on the higher cortical areas (e.g., prefrontal cortex, cingulate cortex, hippocampus, amygdala) as areas critical to development of anxiety. However, the cerebellum is also intimately involved in emotional processing, learning and memory – all of which are represented as risk factors in diathesis models. The following sections will describe how cerebellar activity is related to the signs and symptoms of anxiety and provide often overlooked evidence of cerebellar involvement from imaging research. This will form the basis for speculations regarding individual differences in cerebellar activity as a risk factor for anxiety disorders.

Avoidance. Avoidance is the core feature in the otherwise varied symptomology of anxiety disorders [119]. Therefore, it is essential to understand the role abnormal expressions of avoidance plays in the development and maintenance of anxiety. First, avoidance is acquired and reinforced over time. The essence of anxiety is concern over a potential threatening event in the future, typically one which the individual feels they have no control over and could not cope with. Rather than deal with uncontrollable events, anxious individuals choose to exert their control by substituting other negative thoughts or feelings that are avoidable, providing short term relief and a feeling of temporary control. Avoidance can either be active or passive. In active avoidance, the individual learns to control their environment by alleviating or removing a noxious stimulus. In passive avoidance, the individual learns not to place themselves in a situation that previously contained a noxious stimulus. In anxiety, both forms of avoidance are present, and over time, become pervasive and uncontrollable such that normal functioning becomes impossible.

Avoidance is a learned process. Therefore, it is possible to measure the differences in acquisition of the negative reinforcement learning seen in active-avoidance. Differences in the speed and strength of acquisition in active-avoidance may contribute to risk or resiliency. Some individuals may be more susceptible to acquire and repeatedly express active-avoidance behaviors, leading to development of behavioral and cognitive avoidance symptoms associated with anxiety disorders.

Although the cerebellum is typically associated with associative learning using classical conditioning protocols, a cerebellar role in operant learning such as avoidance has also been suggested. For example, lever press avoidance paradigms places a rat in an operant chamber and presents a stimulus (e.g., tone) that precedes and overlaps with an aversive stimulus (e.g., a shock). Over time, the rat learns to make a lever press response to the tone, avoiding the shock. Lesioning the cerebellum prevents acquisition of the avoidance response in this task [120] and in other measures of active-avoidance [121]. Furthermore, cerebellar involvement may play a role in human avoidance as well [122].

Neuropharmacology. Given the role of the cerebellum and associative learning in anxiety vulnerability, it would be useful to consider treatment approaches that target the cerebellum. Among others, the cerebellum maintains a large density of corticotrophin-releasing hormone (CRH) receptors and cannabinoid receptors. Here, we will outline how these receptors relate to anxiety and eyeblink conditioning.

The influence of CRH on various behavioral markers of anxiety demonstrates its role in modulating stress reactivity. CRH has anxiogenic properties, with a dysregulation of CRH systems playing a role in anxiety disorders. The cerebellum contains a high density of CRH1 receptors, the receptor linked to stress responding, anxious behavior and cognitive functioning [123]. The effects of CRH receptor activation have been thoroughly outlined using animal models, including its influence on anxiety (for a review see [124]). For example, an injection of corticotropin releasing factor (CRF), which induces corticosterone release (the animal analog of cortisol), has been shown to decrease open field exploration, time spent in open arms in the elevated plus maze, exploration in novel environments, and social interaction in rats at certain doses. Furthermore, injections of CRF increase startle amplitude, and improve acquisition in both active and passive avoidance paradigms. Additionally, CRH receptors are adaptive to environmental demands, with a variety of stressors upregulating CRH1 receptors specifically, suggesting a relationship to chronic stress that may feed forward into anxiety disorders [125,126]. Eyeblink conditioning is also influenced by CRH, with studies demonstrating facilitated acquisition in trace paradigms of both humans and rats [127-129]. Humans treated with metyrapone, which decreases initial cortisol response to stress (although not long term effects of stress [130], acquired trace eyeblink conditioning faster than placebo treated controls. While there were no acquisition differences between the groups in delay-type conditioning, metyrapone treated individuals were significantly slower to extinguish, a difference not seen in the trace group [128]. Altogether, it appears that stress reactivity in the brain impacts cerebellar functioning and may play a role in modulating learning and memory, feeding into anxious behavior and increased vulnerability to anxiety disorders.

Cannabinoid receptors, which have their highest densities in the frontal cortex and cerebellum, have also been linked to anxiety [131-133]. Low doses of cannabinoid compounds induce anxiolitic effects, with high doses causing anxiety-like reactions in laboratory rats, suggesting interplay between cannabinoid receptor activity and anxiety [134-136]. These findings are in conjunction with subjective reports that exposure to cannabis derivatives can induce feelings of placid relaxation or panic [137]. For example, low doses of a cannabinoid synthetic reduces behaviors linked to stress in rats with high doses of the same drug causing the opposite pattern, inducing anxiety to novelty and increasing corticosterone [135]. Aside from synthetic activation, endogenous cannabinoid receptor activity is related to anxiety as well. Pharmacological blockage of the CB1 cannabinoid receptor increased anxiety-like behaviors in rats including reduced open arm exploration in the elevated plus maze and increased withdrawal-related behaviors [132]. Cannabinoids influence anxiety and have a high density of receptors in the cerebellum, suggesting that cannabinoid receptor activation would influence eyeblink conditioning as well. As such, animal models have demonstrated that CB1 knockout mice demonstrate disrupted eyeblink conditioning [138] In conjunction, humans who report chronic cannabis use (but not at the time of the study) exhibit fewer and poorly timed CRs during delay eyeblink conditioning compared to non-users [139].

Temperament differences contributes to anxiety vulnerability

Diathesis models suggest that the interplay between risk factors increases vulnerability to develop anxiety disorders. Personality is among the many risk factors suggested to play a role in anxiety, with certain personality types at increased risk to develop anxiety disorders. Support for a personality risk factor in anxiety is supported by the low success rates in treating anxiety disorders, which would require the alteration of stable character traits. Of the few studies that have assessed long-term treatment outcomes of anxiety disorders, 30%-50% still have moderate to severe anxiety six years post treatment [140,141].

An understanding of how personality interacts with anxiety is essential. Here, we will discuss an innate feature of personality known as temperament. Temperament is a core feature of personality, often evident early in childhood and remains stable throughout the lifespan. By measuring temperaments related to anxiety such as behavioral inhibition (BI) and trait anxiety, we are able to differentiate at-risk individuals and assess individual differences on cerebellar modulated tasks.

Behavioral inhibition. Similar to anxiety disorders, a core feature of behavioral inhibition is avoidance. Additionally, the behavioral and physiological functioning of an individual with behavioral inhibition is comparable to that seen in anxiety including withdrawal, apprehension, and slow latency to approach unfamiliar people or objects [142]. Kagan and colleagues have provided an extensive behavioral profile of BI using longitudinal methods, reporting that children classified as inhibited at 21-months demonstrate avoidance of social interactions [143], reported more phobias, and had a higher incidence of anxiety disorders [144-147]. As with anxiety disorders, it appears that inhibited temperament is a heritable trait [148]. Parents and siblings of those children classified as inhibited were more likely to have anxiety disorders, social phobia, avoidant and overanxious disorders compared to the families of uninhibited children [149-151].

So far, we have provided evidence supporting that cerebellar differences underlie higher cognitive processes including anxiety disorders. We have outlined the essential role avoidance has in the development and maintenance of anxiety disorders and how learning processes may underlie increased avoidance. We then introduced behaviorally inhibited temperament, a risk factor with many similarities to anxiety. In the next section we will combine individual differences in cerebellar functioning, avoidance, learning, and temperament to provide a cerebellar diathesis theory of anxiety vulnerability.

As described above, avoidance in the development of anxiety disorders is a feed-forward process, such that the expression of avoidance reduces stress in the present while simultaneously increasing the aversiveness of the undesired stimulus or state in the future, increasing the likelihood of continued avoidance behaviors. Both adaptive and pathological avoidance can be described in terms of the degree and rigidity of expression, the sensitivity to acquire stimulus to stimulus associations, and inflexibility to change. Multiple processes underlie avoidance acquisition, making it difficult to tease out the essential factors in anxiety. It is possible that increased sensitivity to the cues and contingencies in the environment are learned faster in anxiety, resulting in better performance on avoidance tasks. One way to measure these associations is through the classically conditioned eyeblink response. The use of eyeblink conditioning allows multiple measures to be taken into account including reactivity, acquisition of the relationship between the CS and US, and rate of extinction.

Learning. The inbred Wistar-Kyoto rat (WKY) provides a model of inherent anxiousness and vulnerability to stress, similar to what is seen in a behaviorally inhibited personality profile [152-160]. Furthermore, the WKY demonstrates enhanced active avoidance in lever-press paradigms, reinforcing the relationship between anxiety vulnerability and avoidance [161,162]. Comparisons of WKY male rats to outbred Sprague-Dawley male rats demonstrate significantly faster acquisition and greater asymptotic performance of the WKY [163,164]. Moreover, avoidance perseverates in WKY during extinction training in the presence of safety signals [159] or avoidance acquisition with more intense stressors [165]. As reviewed by Jiao [166], the WKY provides an animal model of inhibited temperament, faster associative learning, enhanced sensitivity to acquire avoidance, and resistance to extinction. Moreover, the reactivity increases in the face of avoidance acquisition, reminiscent of increased reactivity in PTSD [167].

Striking parallels are evident between rat models of anxiety vulnerable temperament and humans with self-reported inhibited temperament, suggesting a common neural substrate. One way to assess at-risk temperament is through self-report scales such as those that measure behavioral inhibition [168,169] or trait anxiety [170]. Using these measures, our lab has found that at-risk individuals acquire the relationship between the CS and US the faster, demonstrating more CRs earlier in the training period than those who are low scoring [171,172]. For example, a recent study with a large sample of 117 healthy college-age students found that those scoring high on the Adult Measure of Behavioural Inhibition [169] and Trait Anxiety [170] acquired standard delay eyeblink conditioning faster than those who scored below the median on these measures (see Figure 2). Considering the intimate relationship between associative learning of cues as predictors of aversive events, enhanced classical conditioning may reflect increased sensivity to acquire avoidance responses.

These and other similar results [171,173,174] suggest that individual differences in acquisition of learning tasks may reflect processes underlying increased risk for anxiety disorders.

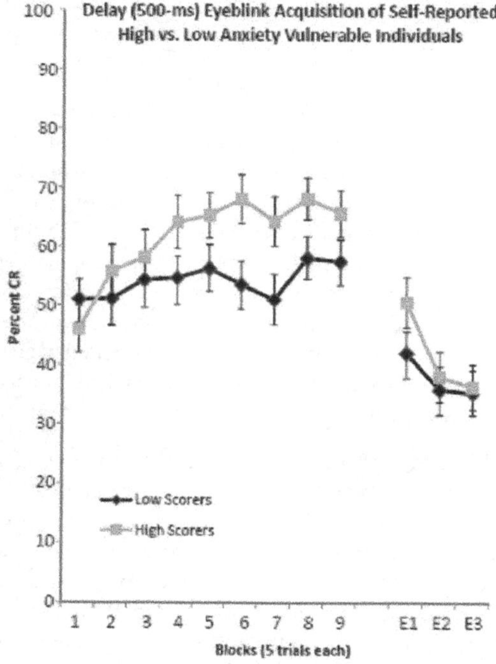

Figure 2. A comparison of temperament on delay eyeblink acquisition of healthy college-aged students. Those who score above the median on the AMBI and STAI-Trait are considered high scorers, those below are considered low scorers Anxiety vulnerable individuals acquired eyeblink conditioning faster and to a greater degree over the 45 trial training period (blocks 1-9). There were no observed differences in extinction (E1-E3).

Heart Rate. In addition to higher cortical pathways, the cerebellum also has direct reciprocal connections to the hypothalamus. Studies in rats and primates show projections from the deep cerebellar nuclei to the lateral hypothalamus, posterior hypothalamic area, dorsal hypothalamic area, the paraventricular nucleus, and the dorsomedial hypothalamic nucleus (For a review see [175]), some of which may be related to heart rate reactivity.

Research in behaviorally inhibited children indicate that a high and stable heart rate (compared to uninhibited children) is indicative of long-term inhibited temperament. Reduced resting heart rate variability has been revealed as a feature of perceived stress [176] and anxiety disorders such as PTSD [177]. The presentation of novel or negative stimuli in healthy populations results in large bradycardic response, with greater bradycardia to more negatively valenced images [178,179]. While there appears to be a relationship between heart rate and anxiety, few studies have looked at heart rate reactivity in behaviorally inhibited adults. Studies that manipulate heart rate typically do so with negatively valenced pictures, assessing reactivity to extreme stimuli (i.e., trauma images for a PTSD patient). In order to disentangle individual reactivity from heart rate changes during high-arousal image processing, which can cause large responses in everyone, a recent study from our lab assessed heart rate change in high and low BI individuals when viewing images that were low in arousal across positive negative and neutral valence. Using this design, we could better understand how BI influences reactivity to everyday stimuli normally encountered in the environment to see if inhibition is related to aberrant parasympathetic or sympathetic activation. Recordings of 6 seconds before, 6 seconds during, and 6 seconds after image presentation suggest a sustained bradycardia in inhibited individuals compared to their non-inhibited counterparts. It is possible that greater vagal tone in high BI could also be related to the enhanced eyeblink acquisition seen in behaviorally inhibited individuals in across studies in Veterans, high school aged students, as well as college aged individuals (See Figure 3).

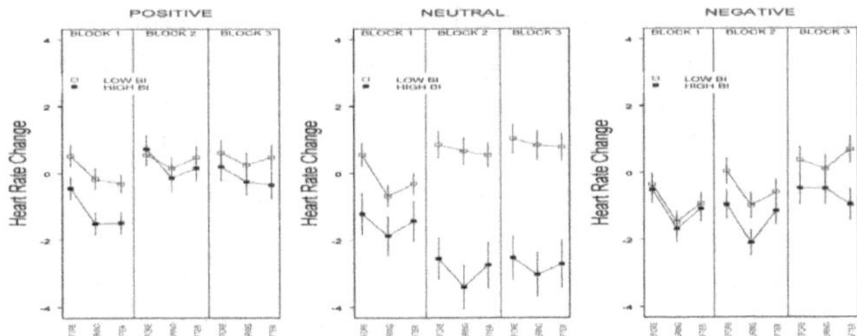

Figure 3. Heart rate change from baseline for positive, neutral, and negative images in high and low behavioral inhibition. Each block represents 20 trials. Behaviorally inhibited individuals showed sutained bradycardia over the neutral picture viewing session. Bradycardia lasted only through the first block of 20 trials in the positive condition, and appeared in the second block (trials 21-40) in the negative condition.

Cerebellar reactivity. Despite being largely ignored and generally not discussed, imaging studies repeatedly indicate significant changes in cerebellar activity of patients with anxiety disorders compared to healthy controls. Close examination of the reported data reveals significant changes in the cerebellum during resting state and anxiety-provoking tasks in social anxiety disorder [180-182], post-traumatic stress disorder [183-187], obsessive compulsive disorder [188] and generalized anxiety disorder [189,190].

Individual differences in cerebellar reactivity have recently been extended to include anxiety vulnerability. Numerous studies assess the correlation between measures of anxiety vulnerability, most often trait anxiety, and brain activity [191]. Mostly, these studies report that individual differences in amygdala and PFC activity underlies trait anxiety, modulating stimulus processing and increasing hypervigilance [192-195]. What is often overlooked is that reciprocal connections between the cerebellum, prefrontal cortex, and amygdala position the cerebellum to modulate reactivity in anxiety vulnerable individuals. In the only published study to date to our knowledge that discusses cerebellar activity and temperament, Blackford and colleagues [10] compared behaviorally inhibited to uninhibited individuals when viewing familiar and novel faces and found significant increases in BOLD activation in the right cerebellum of the inhibited individuals when viewing novel faces. Specifically, they reported significant increases in the right Crus 1/Lobule VI region of the cerebellum, which may be related to processing the valence of emotional cues, salience detection, and in sensory processing and expectation; especially pain-related processes like fear and startle reactions [2,11,76].

The cerebellar differences found in the Blackford study were the result of a full-brain analysis; importantly, standard imaging procedures often incompletely image the cerebellum, so it is possible that the entire structure is not included in typical analyses. Recent research in our lab has explored the relationship of cerebellar activity and anxious temperament as measured by behavioral inhibition and trait anxiety. To extend the Blackford study we again used familiar faces and novel faces. Additionally, we used familiar and novel scenes, allowing us to differentiate the effect of social stimuli and novelty. Furthermore, we used the cerebellum as our region of interest, ensuring complete coverage during imaging. Finally, participants underwent eyeblink conditioning in addition to imaging (outside of the scanner). Given what is known about the behavioral profile of behaviorally inhibited individuals and in light of previous research, we hypothesized that high behavioral inhibition would correlate with changes in cerebellar activity, with the strongest differences occurring to novel faces. We found that the group with higher scores on measures of behavioral inhibition [168,169] had greater cerebellar reactivity to the novel faces compared to baseline than those with lower scores, a difference not seen with familiar faces. Additionally, we observed greater activity of the high BI group when viewing novel scenes, suggesting that the cerebellum may be sensitive to novel stimuli in general. Differences in percent signal change and BOLD signal activations can be seen in figure 4. In eyeblink conditioning, individuals with high BI scores acquired delay eyeblink faster than those with low scores, replicating previous work in our lab.

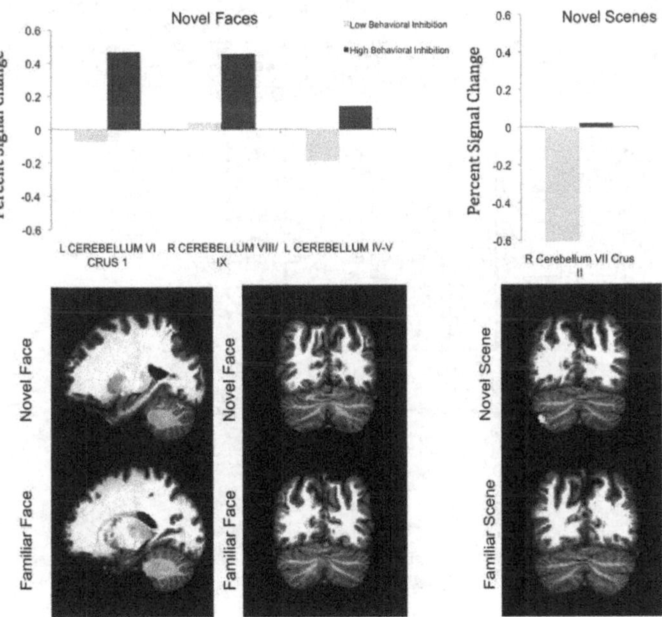

Figure 4. Increased cerebellar reactivity to novel stimuli in anxiety vulnerable individuals. Healthy, college-aged students who scored high on measures of behavioral inhibition demonstrated increased reactivity to multiple areas of the cerebellum in response to novel faces compared to baseline. A similar differential increase in activity was seen for novel scenes. Significant differences in cerebellar activity from baseline were not seen in the familiar face or familiar scene conditions. Left is Right.

We have demonstrated individual differences in cerebellar reactivity and behavior in cerebellar-modulated tasks related to anxiety and anxiety vulnerability. By modulating the signal from higher cortical areas, the cerebellum may be involved in processes related to emotion and anxiety. Figure 5 outlines the cerebrocerebellar and corticopontinecerebellar circuitry as well as the cerebellar outputs for eyeblink conditioning, heart rate responsivity, and higher cognitive process. Cerebellar outputs to prefrontal regions such as the DLPFC and ACC would allow it to modulate incoming signals to these areas regarding higher cognitive functioning including emotion and anxiety. The anatomical pathways, functional connectivity, and individual differences observed of both clinical anxiety and anxiety vulnerable individuals suggest a cerebellar role in anxiety disorders. We propose that cerebellar functioning is another risk factor that needs to be added to the diathesis of anxiety vulnerability. Continued research of individual differences in both cerebellar-modulated tasks (e.g., eyeblink) and the cerebellar role in higher cognitive tasks (e.g., stimulus processing, attention; emotional regulation) will shed light on the interplay of vulnerabilities contributing to the development of anxiety disorders.

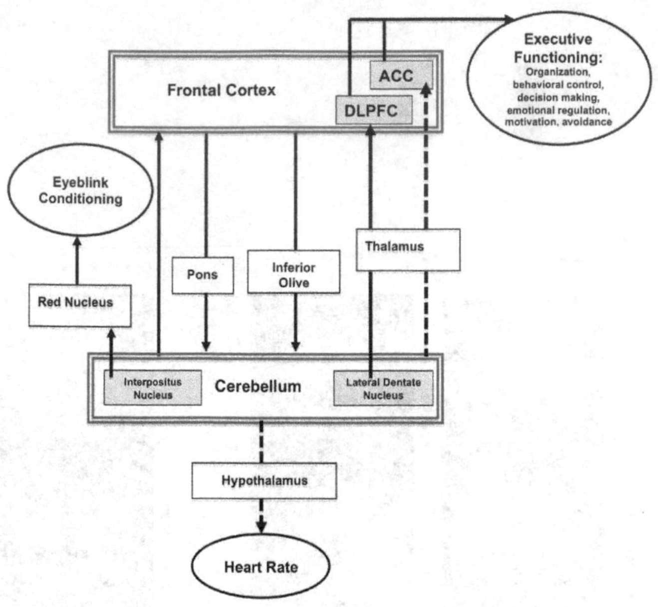

Figure 5. Cerebellar functional connectivity. Reciprocal connectivity with the cortex puts the cerebellum in a position to modulate higher cognitive processes via connections with the dorsolateral prefrontal cortex (DLPFC) and anterior cingulate cortex (ACC). Many functions altered by at-risk temperament may be modulated by the cerebellum including eyeblink conditioning, heart rate reactivity, and executive functioning such as emotional regulation, motivation and avoidance.

Author details

Meghan D. Caulfield and Richard J. Servatius*

*Address all correspondence to: Richard.Servatius@va.gov

Stress & Motivated Behavior Institute, New Jersey Medical School, New Jersey, U. S. A.

References

[1] Gao, H. J., Parsons, L. M., Bower, J. M., Xiong, J., Li, J., & Fox, P. T. (1996). Cerebellum implicated in sensory acquisition and discrimination rather than motor control. *Science.*, 272(5261), 545-7.

[2] Parsons, L. M., Denton, D., Egan, G., Mc Kinley, M., Shade, R., Lancaster, J., et al. (2000). Neuroimaging evidence implicating cerebellum in support of sensory/cognitive processes associated with thirst. *Proceedings of the National Academy of Sciences*, 97(5), 2332-36.

[3] Akshoomoff, N. A., & Courchesne, E. (1992). A new role for the cerebellum in cognitive operations. *Behavioral Neuroscience*, 106(5), 731-8.

[4] Moberget, T., Karns, C. M., Deouell, L. Y., Lindgren, M., Knight, R. T., & Ivry, R. B. (2008). Detecting violations of sensory expectancies following cerebellar degeneration: A mismatch negativity study. *Neuropsychologia*, 46, 2569-79.

[5] Hayter, A. L., & Langdon, D. W. (2007). Cerebellar contributions to working memory. *Neuroimage*, 36(3), 943-54.

[6] Kirschen, M. P., Annabel, Chen. S. H., & Desmond, J. E. (2010). Modality specific cerebro-cerebellar activations in verbal working memory: An fMRI study. *Behavioural Neurology*, 23(1-2), 51-63.

[7] Marvel, C. L., & Desmond, J. E. (2010). topography of the cerebellum in verbal working memory. *Neuropsychology Review*, 20(3), 271-9.

[8] Marvel, C. L., & Desmond, J. E. (2010). The contributions of cerebro-cerebellar circuitry to executive verbal working memory. *Cortex*, 46(7), 880-95.

[9] Liotti, M., Mayberg, H. S., Brannan, S. K., & Mc Ginnis, S. (2000). Differential limbic-cortical correlates of sadness and anxiety in healthy subjects: implications for affective disorders. *Biological Psychiatry*, 48(1), 30-42.

[10] Blackford, J. U., Avery, S. N., Shelton, R. C., & Zald, D. H. (2009). Amygdala temporal dynamics: temperamental differences in the timing of amygdala response to familiar and novel faces. *BMC Neuroscience*, 10(1), 145.

[11] Habas, C., Kamdar, N., Nguyen, D., Prater, K., Beckmann, C. F., Menon, V., et al. (2009). Distinct cerebellar contributions to intrinsic connectivity networks. *Journal of Neuroscience*, 29(26), 8586-94.

[12] Ellis, R. S. (1920). A quantitative study of the purkinje cells in human cerebella. *The Journal of Nervous and Mental Disease*, 51(6), 576.

[13] Ghez, C., & Thach, W. T. The cerebellum. *Kandel ER, Schwartz JH, Jessel TM, editors. Principles of Neural Science. 4th ed. New York: McGraw-HIll*, 832-852.

[14] Apps, R., & Hawkes, R. (2009). Cerebellar cortical organization: a one-map hypothesis. *Nature Reviews Neuroscience*, 10(9), 670-81.

[15] Brooks, V. B., & Thach, T. W. (2011). Cerebellar control of posture and movement. *Comprehensive Physiology*.

[16] Ito, M. (1984). The cerebellum and neural motor control. *New York: Raven*.

[17] Houk, J. C., Keifer, J., & Barto, A. G. (1993). Distributed motor commands in the limb premotor network. *Trends in Neurosciences*, 16(1), 27-33.

[18] Holmes, G. (1939). The cerebellum of man. *Brain*, 62(1), 1-30.

[19] Victor, M., & Adams, R. D. (1959). A restricted form of cerebellar cortical degeneration occurring in alcoholic patients. *Archives of Neurology*, 1(6), 579-688.

[20] Dichgans, J. (1996). Cerebellar and spinocerebellar gait disorders. *In Bronstein AM, Brant T, Woollacott M, eds: Clinical Disorders of Balance Posture and Gait. London: Hodder Arnold Publishers*, 147-155.

[21] Morton, S. M., & Bastian, A. J. (2004). Cerebellar control of balance and locomotion. *Neuroscientist*, 10(3), 247-59.

[22] Fredericks, C. M. (1996). Disorders of the cerebellum and its connections. *In Fredericks CM, Saladin LK. eds: Pathophysiology of the Motor Systems: Principles and Clinical Presentations. FA Davis Co.*

[23] Ivry, R., & Keele, S. (1988). Dissociation of the lateral and medial cerebellum in movement timing and movement execution. *Exp Brain Res*, 73-167.

[24] Ivry, R., & Keele, S. (1989). Timing functions of the cerebellum. *Journal of Cognitive Neuroscience*, 1(2), 136-52.

[25] Bloedel, J. R., Bracha, V., & Larson, P. S. (1993). Real time operations of the cerebellar cortex. *Canadian Journal of Neurological Sciences*, 20(3), S7-18.

[26] Raymond, J. L., & Lisberger, S. G. (1996). The cerebellum: a neuronal learning machine? *Science*, 272, 1126-1131.

[27] Mauk, M. D., Medina, J. F., Nores, W. L., & Ohyama, T. (2000). Cerebellar function: coordination, learning or timing? *Current Biology*, 10(14), R522-5.

[28] Witt, S. T., Laird, A. R., & Meyerand, M. E. (2008). Functional neuroimaging correlates of finger-tapping task variations: an ALE meta-analysis. *Neuroimage*, 42(1), 343-56.

[29] Jueptner, M., Rijntjes, M., Weiller, C., Faiss, J. H., Timmann, D., Mueller, S. P., et al. (1995). Localization of a cerebellar timing process using PET. *Neurology*, 45(8), 1540-5.

[30] O'Reilly, J. X., Mesulam, M. M., & Nobre, A. C. (2008). The cerebellum predicts the timing of perceptual events. *The Journal of Neuroscience*, 28(9), 2252-60.

[31] Koch, G., Oliveri, M., Torriero, S., Salerno, S., Gerfo, Lo. E., & Caltagirone, C. (2007). Repetitive TMS of cerebellum interferes with millisecond time processing. *Experimental Brain Research*, 179(2), 291-9.

[32] Mostofsky, S. H., Kunze, J. C., Cutting, L. E., Lederman, H. M., & Denckla, M. B. (2000). Judgment of duration in individuals with ataxia-telangiectasia. *Developmental Neuropsychology*, 17(1), 63-74.

[33] Hetherington, R., Dennis, M., & Spiegler, B. (2000). Perception and estimation of time in long-term survivors of childhood posterior fossa tumors. *Journal of the International Neuropsychological Society*, 6(6), 682-692.

[34] Malapani, C., Dubois, B., Rancurel, G., & Gibbon, J. (1998). Cerebellar dysfunctions of temporal processing in the seconds range in humans. *Neuroreport*, 9(17), 3907-12.

[35] Ivry, R. B. (1991). Impaired velocity perception in patients with lesions of the cerebellum. *Journal of Cognitive Neuroscience*, 3(4), 355-66.

[36] Nawrot, M., & Rizzo, M. (1995). Motion perception deficits from midline cerebellar lesions in human. *Vision Research*, 35(5), 723-31.

[37] Kent, R. D., Netsell, R., & Abbs, J. H. (1979). Acoustic characteristics of dysarthria associated with cerebellar disease. *Journal of Speech and Hearing Research*, 22(3), 627-48.

[38] Gentil, M. (1990). Dysarthria in Friedreich disease. *Brain and Language*, 38(3), 438-48.

[39] Gentil, M. (1990). EMG analysis of speech production of patients with Friedreich disease. *Clinical Linguistics & Phonetics*, 4(2), 107-20.

[40] Ackermann, H. (1993). Dysarthria in Friedreich's ataxia: timing of speech segments. *Clinical linguistics & Phonetics*, 7(1), 75-91.

[41] Ackermann, H., Hertrich, I., Daum, I., Scharf, G., & Spieker, S. (1997). Kinematic analysis of articulatory movements in central motor disorders. *Movement Disorders*, 12(6), 1019-27.

[42] Swain, R. A., & Thompson, R. F. (1993). In search of engrams. *Annals of the New York Academy of Sciences*, 702, 27-39.

[43] Thompson, R. F., & Kim, J. J. (1996). Memory systems in the brain and localization of a memory. *Proceedings of the National Academy of Sciences*, 93(24), 13438-44.

[44] Thompson, R. F., Bao, S., Chen, L., Cipriano, B. D., Grethe, J. S., Kim, J. J., et al. (1997). Associative learning. *International Review of Neurobiology*, 41, 151-89.

[45] Christian, K. M., & Thompson, R. F. (2003). Neural Substrates of Eyeblink Conditioning: Acquisition and Retention. *Learning & Memory*, 10(6), 427-55.

[46] Thompson, R. F. (1976). The search for the engram. *American Psychologist*, 31(3), 209-27.

[47] Mc Cormick, D. A. (1981). The engram found? Role of the cerebellum in classical conditioning of nictitating membrane and eyelid responses. *Bulletin of the Psychonomic Society*, 18(3), 32, 103-5.

[48] Solomon, P., Stowe, G., & Pendlebeury, W. W. (1989). Disrupted eyelid conditioning in a patient with damage to cerebellar afferents. *Behavioral Neuroscience*, 103(4), 898-902.

[49] Daum, I., Schugens, M., Ackermann, H., Lutzenberger, W., Dichgans, J., & Birbaumer, N. (1993). Classical conditioning after cerebellar lesions in humans. *Behavioral Neuroscience*, 107(5), 748-56.

[50] Topka, H., Valls-Solé, J., Massaquoi, S., & Hallett, M. (1993). Deficit in classical conditioning in patients with cerebellar degeneration. *Brain*, 116, 961-9.

[51] Sears, L. L., & Steinmetz, J. E. (1990). Acquisition of classically conditioned-related activity in the hippocampus is affected by lesions of the cerebellar interpositus nucleus. *Behavioral Neuroscience*, 104(5), 681-92.

[52] Steinmetz, J. E., Lavond, D. G., Ivkovich, D., Logan, C. G., & Thompson, R. F. (1992). Disruption of classical eyelid conditioning after cerebellar lesions: damage to a memory trace system or a simple performance deficit? *The Journal of Neuroscience*, 12(11), 4403-26.

[53] Ivkovich, D., Lockard, J. M., & Thompson, R. F. (1993). Interpositus lesion abolition of the eyeblink conditioned response is not due to effects on performance. *Behavioral Neuroscience*, 107(3), 530-2.

[54] Steinmetz, J. E. (2000). Brain substrates of classical eyeblink conditioning: a highly localized but also distributed system. *Behavioural Brain Research*, 110, 13-24.

[55] Mc Cormick, D. A., Clark, G. A., Lavond, D. G., & Thompson, R. F. (1982). Initial localization of the memory trace for a basic form of learning. *Proceedings of the National Academy of Sciences*, 79(8), 2731-5.

[56] Mc Cormick, D. A., & Thompson, R. F. (1984). Cerebellum: essential involvement in the classically conditioned eyelid response. *Science*, 223(4633), 296-9.

[57] Thompson, R. F. (1986). The neurobiology of learning and memory. *Science*, 233(4767), 941-47.

[58] Rosenfield, M. E., & Moore, J. W. (1983). Red nucleus lesions disrupt the classically conditioned nictitating membrane response in rabbits. *Behavioural Brain Research*, 10(2-3), 393-8.

[59] Rosenfield, M. E., & Moore, J. W. (1985). Red nucleus lesions impair acquisition of the classically conditioned nictitating membrane response but not eye-to-eye savings or unconditioned response amplitude. *Behavioural Brain Research*, 17(1), 77-81.

[60] Schugens, M. M., Egerter, R., Daum, I., Schepelmann, K., Kockgether, T., & Loschmann, P. A. (1997). The NMDA antagonist memantine impairs classical eyeblink conditioning in humans. *Neuroscience Letters*, 224, 57-60.

[61] Logan, C. G., & Grafton, S. T. (1995). Functional anatomy of human eyeblink conditioning determined with regional cerebral glucose metabolism and positron-emission tomography. *Proceedings of the National Academy of Sciences*, 92(16), 7500-4.

[62] Blaxton, T. A., Zeffiro, T. A., Gabrieli, J. D. E., Bookheimer, S. Y., Carrillo, M. C., Theodore, W. H., et al. (1996). Functional mapping of human learning: A positron emis-

sion tomography activation study of eyeblink conditioning. *The Journal of Neuroscience*, 16(12), 4032-40.

[63] Knuttinen, M. G., Parrish, T. B., Weiss, C., La Bar, K. S., Gitelman, D. R., Power, J. M., et al. (2002). Electromyography as a recording system for eyeblink conditioning with functional magnetic resonance imaging. *Neuroimage*, 17(2), 977-87.

[64] Knight, D. C., Cheng, D. T., Smith, C. N., Stein, E. A., & Helmstetter, F. J. (2004). Neural substrates mediating human delay and trace fear conditioning. *The Journal of Neuroscience*, 24(1), 218-28.

[65] Cheng, D. T., Disterhoft, J. F., Power, J. M., Ellis, D. A., & Desmond, J. E. (2008). Neural substrates underlying human delay and trace eyeblink conditioning. *Proceedings of the National Academy of Sciences*, 105(23), 8108-13.

[66] Mc Glinchey-Berroth, R., Cermak, L. S., Carrillo, M. C., Armfield, S., & Gabrieli, Disterhoft. J. F. (1995). Impaired delay eyeblink conditioning in amnesic Korsakoff's patients and recovered alcoholics. *Alcoholism, Clinical and Experimental Research*, 19(5), 1127-32.

[67] Coffin, J. M., Baroody, S., Schneider, K., & O'Neill, J. (2005). Impaired cerebellar learning in children with prenatal alcohol exposure: a comparative study of eyeblink conditioning in children with ADHD and dyslexia. *Cortex*, 41(3), 389-98.

[68] Jacobson, S. W., Stanton, M. E., Molteno, C. D., Burden, M. J., Fuller, D. S., Hoyme, H. E., et al. (2008). Impaired eyeblink conditioning in children with fetal alcohol syndrome. *Alcoholism, Clinical and Experimental Research*, 32(2), 365-72.

[69] Jacobson, S. W., Stanton, M. E., Dodge, N. C., Pienaar, M., Fuller, D. S., Molteno, C. D., et al. (2011). Impaired delay and trace eyeblink conditioning in school-age children with fetal alcohol syndrome. *Alcoholism, Clinical and Experimental Research*, 35(2), 250-64.

[70] Sears, L. L., Finn, P. R., & Steinmetz, J. E. (1994). Abnormal classical eye-blink conditioning in autism. *Journal of Autism and Developmental Disorders*, 24(6), 737-51.

[71] Steinmetz, L. (2000). Classical eyeblink conditioning in normal and autistic children. *Eyeblink classical conditioning*, I, 143-162.

[72] Sears, L. L., Andreasen, N. C., & O'Leary, D. S. (2000). Cerebellar functional abnormalities in schizophrenia are suggested by classical eyeblink conditioning. *Biological Psychiatry*, 48(3), 204-9.

[73] Cartford, M. C., & Gemma, C. (2002). Eighteen-month-old Fischer 344 rats fed a spinach-enriched diet show improved delay classical eyeblink conditioning and reduced expression of tumor necrosis. *The Journal of Neuroscience*, 22(14), 5813-6.

[74] Courchesne, E., & Allen, G. (1997). Prediction and preparation, fundamental functions of the cerebellum. *Learning & Memory*, 4(1), 1-35.

[75] Schmahmann, J. D. (1996). From Movement to Thought: Anatomic Substrates of the Cerebellar Contribution to Cognitive Processing. *Human Brain Mapping*, 4, 174-98.

[76] Stoodley, C., & Schmahmann, J. (2009). Functional topography in the human cerebellum: A meta-analysis of neuroimaging studies. *Neuroimage*, 44(2), 489-501.

[77] Strick, P. L., Dum, R. P., & Fiez, J. A. (2009). Cerebellum and nonmotor function. *Annual Review of Neuroscience*, 32, 413-34.

[78] Desmond, J. E., & Fiez, J. A. (1998). Neuroimaging studies of the cerebellum: Language, learning and memory. *Trends in Cognitive Sciences*, 2(9), 355-62.

[79] Steinlin, M. (2007). The cerebellum in cognitive processes: Supporting studies in children. *The cerebellum*, 6(3), 237-41.

[80] Brodal, P., Bjaalie, J. G., & Aas, J. E. (1991). Organization of cingulo-ponto-cerebellar connections in the cat. *Anatomy and Embryology*, 184(3), 245-54.

[81] Middleton, F. A., & Strick, P. L. (1994). Anatomical evidence for cerebellar and basal ganglia involvement in higher cognitive function. *Science*, 266(5184), 458-61.

[82] Schmahmann, J. D., & Pandya, D. N. (1995). Prefrontal cortex projections to the basilar pons in rhesus monkey: implications for the cerebellar contribution to higher function. *Neuroscience Letters*, 199, 175-8.

[83] Middleton, F. A., & Strick, P. L. (1997). Cerebellar output channels. *International Review of Neurobiology*, 41, 61-82.

[84] Middleton, F. A., & Strick, P. L. (2001). Cerebellar projections to the prefrontal cortex of the primate. *The Journal of Neuroscience*, 21(2), 700-12.

[85] Kelly, R. M., & Strick, P. L. (2003). Cerebellar loops with motor cortex and prefrontal cortex of a nonhuman primate. *The Journal of Neuroscience*, 23(23), 8432-44.

[86] Fuster, J. M. (2000). Executive frontal functions. *Experimental Brain Research*, 133, 66-70.

[87] Bor, D., Duncan, J., Wiseman, R. J., & Owen, A. M. (2003). Encoding strategies dissociate prefrontal activity from working memory demand. *Neuron*, 37(2), 361-7.

[88] Goldman-Rakic, P. S. (1987). Circuitry of primate prefrontal cortex and regulation of behavior by representational memory. *CComprehensive Physiology*.

[89] Postle, B. R., Berger, J. S., Taich, A. M., & D'Esposito, M. (2000). Activity in human frontal cortex associated with spatial working memory and saccadic behavior. *Journal of Cognitive Neuroscience*, 2, 2-14.

[90] Damasio, A. R. (1995). On Some Functions of the Human Prefrontal Cortex. *Annals of the New York Academy of Sciences*, 769, 241-52.

[91] Li, J., Delgado, M. R., & Phelps, E. A. (2011). How instructed knowledge modulates the neural systems of reward learning. . *Proceedings of the National Academy of Sciences*, 108(1), 55-60.

[92] Hikosaka, K., & Watanabe, M. (2004). Long- and short-range reward expectancy in the primate orbitofrontal cortex. *European Journal of Neuroscience*, 19(4), 1046-54.

[93] Dum, R. P., & Strick, P. L. (2002). An Unfolded Map of the Cerebellar Dentate Nucleus and its Projections to the Cerebral Cortex. *Journal of Neurophysiology*, 89(1), 634-9.

[94] Allen, G., Mc Coll, R., Barnard, H., Ringe, W. K., Fleckenstein, J., & Cullum, C. M. (2005). Magnetic resonance imaging of cerebellar-prefrontal and cerebellar-parietal functional connectivity. *Neuroimage*, 28, 39-48.

[95] Yan, H., Zuo-N, X., Wang, D., Wang, J., Zhu, C., Milham, M. P., et al. (2009). Hemispheric asymmetry in cognitive division of anterior cingulate cortex: a resting-state functional connectivity study. *Neuroimage*, 47(4), 1579-89.

[96] Schmahmann, J. D., Macmore, J, & Vangel, M. (2009). Cerebellar stroke without motor deficit: clinical evidence for motor and non-motor domains within the human cerebellum. *Neuroscience*, 162(3), 852-61.

[97] Schmahmann, J. D., & Sherman, J. C. (1998). The cerebellar cognitive affective syndrome. *Brain*, 121(Pt 4), 561-79.

[98] Nobre, A. C., Sebestyen, G. N., & Gitelman, D. R. (1997). Functional localization of the system for visuospatial attention using positron emission tomography. *Brain*, 120(3), 515-33.

[99] Coull, J. T., & Nobre, A. C. (1998). Where and when to pay attention: the neural systems for directing attention to spatial locations and to time intervals as revealed by both PET and fMRI. *The Journal of Neuroscience*, 18(18), 7426-35.

[100] Kim, Y. H., Gitelman, D. R., Nobre, A. C., & Parrish, T. B. (1999). The large-scale neural network for spatial attention displays multifunctional overlap but differential asymmetry. *Neuroimage*, 9(3), 269-77.

[101] La Bar, K. S., Gitelman, D. R., Parrish, T. B., & Mesulam, M. (1999). Neuroanatomic overlap of working memory and spatial attention networks: a functional MRI comparison within subjects. *Neuroimage*, 10(6), 695-704.

[102] Marvel, C. L., & Desmond, J. E. (2010). The contributions of cerebro-cerebellar circuitry to executive verbal working memory. *Cortex*, 46(7), 880-95.

[103] Heath, R. G., & Harper, J. W. (1974). Ascending projections of the cerebellar fastigial nucleus to the hippocampus, amygdala, and other temporal lobe sites: evoked potential and histological studies in monkeys and cats. *Experimental Neurolology*, Jun. 13;, 45, 268-87.

[104] Lee, G. P., Meador, K. J., Loring, D. W., Allison, J. D., Brown, W. S., Paul, L. K., et al. (2004). Neural substrates of emotion as revealed by functional magnetic resonance imaging. *Cognitive Behavioral Neurology*, 17, 9-17.

[105] Bermpohl, F., Pascual-Leone, A., Amedi, A., Merabet, L. B., Fregni, F., Gaab, N., et al. (2006). Dissociable networks for the expectancy and perception of emotional stimuli in the human brain. *Neuroimage*, 30, 588-600.

[106] Hofer, A., Siedentopf, C. M., Ischebeck, A., Rettenbacher, M. A., Verius, M., Felber, S., et al. (2007). Sex differences in brain activation patterns during processing of positively and negatively valenced emotional words. *Psychological Medicine*, 37(1), 109-19.

[107] Berntson, G. G., Potolicchio, S. J., & Miller, N. E. (1973). Evidence for higher functions of the cerebellum: eating and grooming elicited by cerebellar stimulation in cats. *Proceedings of the National Academy of Sciences*, 70(9), 2497-9.

[108] Ball, G. G., Micco, D. J., & Berntson, G. G. (1974). Cerebellar stimulation in the rat: complex stimulation-bound oral behaviors and self-stimulation. *Physiology & Behavior*, 13(1), 123-7.

[109] Watson, P. J. (1978). Nonmotor Functions of the Cerebellum. *Psychological Bulletin*, 85(5), 944-67.

[110] Supple, W. F., Leaton, R. N., & Fanselow, M. S. (1987). Effects of cerebellar vermal lesions on species-specific fear responses, neophobia, and taste-aversion learning in rats. *Physiology & Behavior*, 39(5), 579-86.

[111] Leaton, R. N., & Supple, W. F. (1986). Cerebellar vermis: essential for long-term habituation of the acoustic startle response. *Science*, 232(4749), 513-5.

[112] Heath, R. G., Cox, A. W., & Lustick, L. S. (1974). Brain activity during emotional states. *American Journal of Psychiatry*, 131(8), 858-62.

[113] Blaine, S., Nadhold, J., & Slaughter, D. G. (1969). Effects of stimulating or destroying the deep cerebellar regions in man. *Journal of Neurosurgery*, 31, 172-86.

[114] Cooper, I. S., Amin, I., Riklan, M., Waltz, J. M., Tung, Pui., & Poon, M. D. (1976). Chronic cerebellar stimulation in epilepsy: clinical and anatomical studies. *Archives of Neurology*, 33(8), 559-70.

[115] Rapoport, M., van Reekum, R., & Mayberg, H. (2000). The role of the cerebellum in cognition and behavior: a selective review. *The Journal of Neuropsychiatry and Clinical Neurosciences*, 12(2), 193-8.

[116] Kessler, R. C., Berglund, P., Demler, O., Jin, R., Merikangas, K. R., & Walters, E. E. (2005). Lifetime prevalence and age-of-onset distributions of DSM-IV disorders in the National Comorbidity Survey Replication. *Archives of General Psychiatry*, 62(6), 593-602.

[117] Kessler, R. C., Chiu, W. T., Demler, O., Merikangas, K. R., & Walters, E. E. (2005). Prevalence, severity, and comorbidity of 12-month DSM-IV disorders in the National Comorbidity Survey Replication. *Archives of General Psychiatry*, 62(6), 617-27.

[118] Mineka, S., & Zinbarg, R. (2006). A contemporary learning theory perspective on the etiology of anxiety disorders: It's not what you thought it was. *American Psychologist*, 61(1), 10-26.

[119] American Psychiatric Association. (2000). Diagnostic and statistical manual of mental disorders: DSM IV-TR. 4th ed. American Psychiatric Association. *Washington, DC*.

[120] Steinmetz, J. E., Logue, S. F., & Miller, D. P. (1993). Using signaled barpressing tasks to study the neural substrates of appetitive and aversive learning in rats: behavioral manipulations and cerebellar lesions. *Behavioral Neuroscience*, 107(6), 941-54.

[121] Dahhaoui, M., Caston, J., & Auvray, N. (1990). Role of the cerebellum in an avoidance conditioning task in the rat. *Physiology & Behavior*, 47, 1175-80.

[122] Schlund, M. W., & Cataldo, M. F. (2010). Amygdala involvement in human avoidance, escape and approach behavior. *Neuroimage*, 53(2), 769-76.

[123] Holsboer, F. (1999). The rationale for corticotropin-releasing hormone receptor (CRH-R) antagonists to treat depression and anxiety. *Journal of Psychiatric Research*, 33(3), 181-214.

[124] Dunn, A. J., & Berridge, C. W. (1990). Physiological and behavioral responses to corticotropin-releasing factor administration: is CRF a mediator of anxiety or stress responses. *Brain Research Reviews*, 15(71), 100.

[125] Lacroix, S., & Rivest, S. (1996). Role of cyclo-oxygenase pathways in the stimulatory influence of immune challenge on the transcription of a specific CRF receptor subtype in the rat brain. *Journal of Chemical Neuroanatomy*, 10(1), 53-71.

[126] Giardino, L., Puglisi-Allegra, S., & Ceccatelli, S. (1996). CRH-R1 mRNA expression in two strains of inbred mice and its regulation after repeated restraint stress. *Molecular Brain Research*, 40(2), 310-14.

[127] Servatius, R. J., Beck, K. D., Moldow, R. L., & Salameh, G. (2005). A stress-induced anxious state in male rats: corticotropin-releasing hormone induces persistent changes in associative learning and startle reactivity. *Biological Psychiatry*, 57(1), 865-72.

[128] Nees, F., Richter, S., Lass-Hennemann, J., Blumenthal, T. D., & Schächinger, H. (2008). Inhibition of cortisol production by metyrapone enhances trace, but not delay, eyeblink conditioning. *Psychopharmacology*, 199(2), 183-90.

[129] Kuehl, L. K., Lass-Hennemann, J., Richter, S., Blumenthal, T. D., Oitzl, M., & Schächinger, H. (2010). Accelerated trace eyeblink conditioning after cortisol IV-infusion. *Neurobiology of Learning and Memory*, 94(4), 547-53.

[130] Brennan, F. X., Ottenweller, J. E., & Servatius, R. J. (2001). Pharmacological suppression of corticosterone secretion in response to a physical stressor does not prevent the delayed persistent increase in circulating basal. *Stress*, 4(2), 137-141.

[131] Herkenham, M., Lynn, A. B., Little, M. D., Johnson, M. R., Melvin, L. S., De Costa, B. R., et al. (1990). Cannabinoid receptor localization in brain. *Proceedings of the National Academy of Sciences*, 87(5), 932.

[132] Navarro, M., Hernández, E., Muñoz, R. M., del Arco, I., Villanúa, MA, Carrera, M. R. A., et al. (1997). Acute administration of the CB1 cannabinoid receptor antagonist SR 141716A induces anxiety-like responses in the rat. *Neuroreport*, 8(2), 491-6.

[133] Haller, J., Bakos, N., Szirmay, M., Ledent, C., & Freund, T. F. (2002). The effects of genetic and pharmacological blockade of the CB1 cannabinoid receptor on anxiety. *European Journal of Neuroscience*, 16(7), 1395-8.

[134] Onaivi, E. S., Green, M. R., & Martin, B. R. (1990). Pharmacological characterization of cannabinoids in the elevated plus maze. *Journal of Pharmacology and Experimental Therapeutics*, 253(3), 1002-1009.

[135] de Fonseca, F. R., Rubio, P., Menzaghi, F., Merlo-Pich, E., Rivier, J., Koob, G. F., & Navarro, M. (1996). Corticotropin-releasing factor (CRF) antagonist [D-Phe12, Nle21, 38, C alpha MeLeu37] CRF attenuates the acute actions of the highly potent cannabinoid receptor agonist HU-210 on defensive-withdrawal behavior in rats. *Journal of Pharmacology and Experimental Therapeutics*, 276(1), 56-64.

[136] Navarro, M., Fernández-Ruiz, J. J., De Miguel, R., Hernández, M. L., Cebeira, M., & Ramos, J. A. (1993). An acute dose of delta 9-tetrahydrocannabinol affects behavioral and neurochemical indices of mesolimbic dopaminergic activity. *Behavioural Brain Research*, 57(1), 37-46.

[137] Hollister, L. E. (1986). Health aspects of cannabis. *Pharmacological Reviews*, 38(1), 1-20.

[138] Kishimoto, Y., & Kano, M. (2006). Endogenous cannabinoid signaling through the CB1 receptor is essential for cerebellum-dependent discrete motor learning. *The Journal of Neuroscience*, 26(34), 8829-37.

[139] Skosnik, P. D., Edwards, C. R., O'Donnell, B. F., Steffen, A., Steinmetz, J. E., & Hetrick, W. P. (2008). Cannabis use disrupts eyeblink conditioning: evidence for cannabinoid modulation of cerebellar-dependent learning. *Neuropsychopharmacology*, 33(6), 1432-40.

[140] Noyes, R., Jr., Clancy, J., & Hoenk, P. R. (1980). The prognosis of anxiety neurosis. *Archives of General Psychiatry*, 37(2), 173.

[141] Kendall, P. C., Brady, E. U., & Verduin, T. L. (2001). Comorbidity in childhood anxiety disorders and treatment outcome. *Journal of the American Academy of Child & Adolescent Psychiatry*, 40(7), 787-94.

[142] Garcia Coll, C., & Kagan, J. (1984). Behavioral inhibition in young children. *Child Development*, 55(3), 1005-19.

[143] Kagan, J., & Moss, H. A. (1962). *Birth to maturity: A study in psychological development.*, Yale University Press.

[144] Hirshfeld, D., Rosenbaum, J., & Biederman, J. (1992). Stable Behavioral Inhibition and Its Association with Anxiety Disorder. *Journal of the American Academy of Child & Adolescent Psychiatry*, 31(1), 103-11.

[145] Schwartz, C. E., & Snidman, N. (1999). Adolescent social anxiety as an outcome of inhibited temperament in childhood. *of the American Academy of Child & Adolescent Psychiatry*, 38(8), 1008-15.

[146] Biederman, J., Rosenbaum, J. F., Hirshfeld, D. R., Faraone, S. V., Bolduc, E. A., Gersten, M., et al. (1990). Psychiatric correlates of behavioral inhibition in young children of parents with and without psychiatric disorders. *Archives of General Psychiatry*, 47(1), 21.

[147] Biederman, J., & Hirshfeld-Becker, D. (2001). Further evidence of association between behavioral inhibition and social anxiety in children. *American journal of Psychiatry*, 158(10), 1673-79.

[148] Robinson, J., Kagan, J., & Reznick, J. S. (1992). The heritability of inhibited and uninhibited behavior: A twin study. *Developmental Psychology*, 28(6), 1030-37.

[149] Rosenbaum, J., Biederman, J., & Hirshfeld, D. (1991). Further evidence of an association between behavioral inhibition and anxiety disorders: Results from a family study of children from a non-clinical sample. *Journal of Psychiatric Research*, 25(1), 49-65.

[150] Rosenbaum, J. F., & Biederman, J. (1992). Comorbidity of parental anxiety disorders as risk for childhood-onset anxiety in inhibited children. *The American Journal of Psychiatry*, 149(4), 475-81.

[151] Rosenbaum, J. F., Biederman, J., Hirshfeld-Becker, D. R., Kagan, J., Snidman, N., Friedman, D., et al. (2000). A controlled study of behavioral inhibition in children of parents with panic disorder and depression. *American Journal of Psychiatry*, 157(12), 2002-10.

[152] Paré, W. P. (1989). Strain, age, but not gender, influence ulcer severity induced by water-restraint stress. *Physiology & Behavior*, 45(3), 627-32.

[153] Paré, W. P. (1989). Stress ulcer susceptibility and depression in Wistar Kyoto (WKY) rats. *Physiology & Behavior*, 46(6), 993-8.

[154] Paré, W. P. (1993). Passive-avoidance behavior in Wistar-Kyoto (WKY), Wistar, and Fischer-344 rats. *Physiology & Behavior*, 54(5), 845-52.

[155] Paré, W. P. (1994). Open field, learned helplessness, conditioned defensive burying, and forced-swim tests in WKY rats. *Physiology & Behavior*, 55(3), 433-9.

[156] Redei, E., Paré, W. P., Aird, F., & Kluczynski, J. (1994). Strain differences in hypothalamic-pituitary-adrenal activity and stress ulcer. *American Journal of Physiology-Regulatory, Integrative and Comparative Physiology*, 266(2), R353-60.

[157] Armario, A., Gavaldà, A., & Martí, J. (1995). Comparison of the behavioural and endocrine response to forced swimming stress in five inbred strains of rats. *Psychoneuroendocrinology*, 20(8), 879-90.

[158] Rittenhouse, P. A., López-Rubalcava, C., Stanwood, G. D., & Lucki, I. (2002). Amplified behavioral and endocrine responses to forced swim stress in the Wistar-Kyoto rat. *Psychoneuroendocrinology*, 27(3), 303-18.

[159] Servatius, R. J., Jiao, X., Beck, K. D., Pang, K. C. H., & Minor, T. R. (2008). Rapid avoidance acquisition in Wistar-Kyoto rats. *Behavioural Brain Research*, 192(2), 191-7.

[160] McAuley, J. D., Stewart, A. L., Webber, E. S., Cromwell, H. C., Servatius, R. J., & Pang, K. C. H. (2009). Wistar-Kyoto rats as an animal model of anxiety vulnerability: support for a hypervigilance hypothesis. *Behavioural Brain Research*, 204(1), 162-8.

[161] Servatius, R. J., Jiao, X., Beck, K. D., & Pang, K. (2008). Rapid avoidance acquisition in Wistar-Kyoto rats. *Behavioural Brain Research*, 192(2), 191-97.

[162] Beck, K. D., Jiao, X., Pang, K. C. H., & Servatius, R. J. (2010). Vulnerability factors in anxiety determined through differences in active-avoidance behavior. *Progress in Neuro-Psychopharmacology and Biological Psychiatry*, 34(6), 852-60.

[163] Ricart, T. M., Jiao, X., Pang, K. C. H., Beck, K. D., & Servatius, R. J. (2011). Classical and instrumental conditioning of eyeblink responses in Wistar-Kyoto and Sprague-Dawley rats. *Behavioural Brain Research*, 216(1), 414-8.

[164] Ricart, T. M., De Niear, M. A., Jiao, X., Pang, K. C. H., Beck, K. D., & Servatius, R. J. (2011). Deficient proactive interference of eyeblink conditioning in Wistar-Kyoto rats. *Behavioural Brain Research*, 216(1), 59-65.

[165] Jiao, X., Pang, K. C. H., Beck, K. D., Minor, T. R., & Servatius, R. J. (2011). Avoidance perseveration during extinction training in Wistar-Kyoto rats: an interaction of innate vulnerability and stressor intensity. *Behavioural Brain Research*, 221(1), 98-107.

[166] Jiao, X., Beck, K. D., Pang, K. C. H., & Servatius, R. J. (2011). Animal Models of Anxiety Vulnerability- The Wistar Kyoto Rat. *Selek S, editor. Different View of Anxiety Disorders. Rijeka:InTech.*

[167] Ricart, T. M., Servatius, R. J., & Beck, K. D. (2012). Acquisition of Active Avoidance Behavior as a Precursor to Changes in General Arousal in an Animal Model of PTSD. *Ovuga E, editor. Post Traumatic Stress Disorders in a Global Context. Rijeka: InTech.*

[168] Reznick, J. S., Hegeman, I. M., Kaufman, E. R., Woods, S. W., & Jacobs, M. (1992). Retrospective and concurrent self-report of behavioral inhibition and their relation to adult mental health. *Development and Psychopatholoy*, 4, 301-21.

[169] Gladstone, G., & Parker, G. (2005). Measuring a behaviorally inhibited temperament style: Development and initial validation of new self-report measures. *Psychiatry Research*, 135, 133-43.

[170] Spielberger, C., Gorsuch, R., & Lushene, R. (1970). Spielberger: Manual for the State-Trait Anxiety. *Palo Alto, CA: Consulting Psychologists Press.*

[171] Myers, C. E., Van Meenen, K. M., Mc Auley, J. D., Beck, K. D., Pang, K. C. H., & Servatius, R. J. (2011). Behaviorally inhibited temperament is associated with severity of post-traumatic stress disorder symptoms and faster eyeblink conditioning in veterans. *Stress*, 15(1), 31-44.

[172] Myers, C. E., Van Meenen, K. M., & Servatius, R. J. (2012). Behavioral inhibition and PTSD symptoms in veterans. *Psychiatry Research*, 196(2), 271-6.

[173] Farber, I. E., & Spence, K. W. (1953). Complex learning and conditioning as a function of anxiety. *Journal of Psychology*, 45(2), 120-5.

[174] Spence, K. W., & Beecroft, R. S. (1954). Differential conditioning and level of anxiety. *Journal of Experimental Psychology*, 48(5), 399-403.

[175] Zhu-N, J., Yung-H, W., Kwok-Chong, Chow. B., Chan-S, Y., & Wang-J, J. (2006). The cerebellar-hypothalamic circuits: potential pathways underlying cerebellar involvement in somatic-visceral integration. *Brain Research Reviews*, 52(1), 93-106.

[176] Dishman, R. K., Nakamura, Y., Garcia, M. E., Thompson, R. W., Dunn, A. L., & Blair, S. N. (2000). Heart rate variability, trait anxiety, and perceived stress among physically fit men and women. *International Journal of Psychophysiology*, 37, 121-33.

[177] Cohen, H., Benjamin, J., Geva, A. B., Matar, M. A., Kaplan, Z., & Kotler, M. (2000). Autonomic dysregulation in panic disorder and in post-traumatic stress disorder: application of power spectrum analysis of heart rate variability at rest and in response to recollection of trauma or panic attacks. *Psychiatry Research*, 96(1), 1-13.

[178] Bohlin, G., Graham, F. K., Silverstein, L. D., & Hackley, S. A. (1981). Cardiac orinting and startle blink modification in novel and signal situations. *Psychophysiology*, 18(5), 603-11.

[179] Bradley, M. M., Lang, P. J., & Cuthbert, B. N. (1993). Emotion, Novelty, and the Startle Reflex: Habituation in Humans. *Behavioral neuroscience*, 107(6), 970-80.

[180] Kilts, C. D., Kelsey, J. E., Knight, B., Ely, T. D., Bowman, F. D., Gross, R. E., et al. (2006). The neural correlates of social anxiety disorder and response to pharmacotherapy. *Neuropsychopharmacology*, 31(10), 2243-53.

[181] Evans, K. C., Wright, C. I., Wedig, M. M., Gold, A. L., Pollack, M. H., & Rauch, S. L. (2008). A functional MRI study of amygdala responses to angry schematic faces in social anxiety disorder. *Depression and Anxiety*, 25(6), 496-505.

[182] Warwick, J. M., Carey, P., Jordaan, G. P., Dupont, P., & Stein, D. J. (2008). Resting brain perfusion in social anxiety disorder: a voxel-wise whole brain comparison with

healthy control subjects. *Progress in Neuro-Psychopharmacology and Biological Psychiatry*, 32(5), 1251-6.

[183] Shin, L. M., Mc Nally, R. J., Kosslyn, S. M., Thompson, W. L., Rauch, S. L., Alpert, N. M., et al. (1999). Regional Cerebral Blood Flow During Script-Driven Imagery in Childhood Sexual Abuse-Related PTSD: A PET Investigation. *American Journal of Psychiatry*, 156, 575-84.

[184] Bremner, J. D., Narayan, M., Staib, L. H., Southwick, S. M., Mc Glashan, T., & Charney, D. S. (1999). Neural Correlates of Memories of Childhood Sexual Abuse in Women With and Without Posttraumatic Stress Disorder. *The American journal of psychiatry*, 156, 1787-95.

[185] Bremner, J. D., Vythilingam, M., Vermetten, E., Southwick, S. M., Mc Glashan, T., Staib, L. H., et al. (2003). Neural correlates of declarative memory for emotionally valenced words in women with posttraumatic stress disorder related to early childhood sexual abuse. *Biological Psychiatry*, 53(10), 879-89.

[186] Bonne, O., Gilboa, A., Louzoun, Y., Brandes, D., Yona, I., Lester, H., et al. (2003). Resting regional cerebral perfusion in recent posttraumatic stress disorder. *Biological Psychiatry*, 54(10), 1077-86.

[187] Yang, P., Wu, T. M., Hsu-C, C., & Ker-H, J. (2004). Evidence of early neurobiological alternations in adolescents with posttraumatic stress disorder: a functional MRI study. *Neuroscience Letters*, 370(1), 13-8.

[188] Menzies, L., Achard, S., Chamberlain, S. R., Fineberg, N., Chen-H, C., del Campo, N., et al. (2007). Neurocognitive endophenotypes of obsessive-compulsive disorder. *Brain*, 130(12), 3223-36.

[189] Blair, K., Shaywitz, J., Smith, B. W., et al. (2008). Response to emotional expressions in generalized social phobia and generalized anxiety disorder: evidence for separate disorders. *American Journal of Psychiatry*, 165(9), 1193-1202.

[190] Chen, J. (2011). A review of neuroimaging studies of anxiety disorders in China. *Neuropsychiatric Disease and Treatment*, 7, 241-249.

[191] Schwartz, C. E., & Rauch, S. L. (2004). Temperament and its implications for neuroimaging of anxiety disorders. *CNS Spectrums*, 9(4), 284-91.

[192] Etkin, A., Klemenhagen, K. C., Dudman, J. T., Rogan, M. T., Hen, R., Kandel, E. R., et al. (2004). Individual differences in trait anxiety predict the response of the basolateral amygdala to unconsciously processed fearful faces. *Neuron*, 44, 1043-55.

[193] Bishop, S. J. (2008). Trait anxiety and impoverished prefrontal control of attention. *Nature Neuroscience*, 12(1), 92-98.

[194] Schienle, A., Schäfer, A., Stark, R., Walter, B., & Vaitl, D. (2005). Relationship between disgust sensitivity, trait anxiety and brain activity during disgust induction. *Neuropsychobiology*, 51(2), 86-92.

[195] Blackford, J. U., Avery, S. N., Cowan, R. L., Shelton, R. C., & Zald, D. H. (2010). Sustained amygdala response to both novel and newly familiar faces characterizes inhibited temperament. *Social Cognitive and Affective Neuroscience*, 6(5), 621-9.

Chapter 5

Alterations in the Immune Response, Apoptosis and Synaptic Plasticity in Posttraumatic Stress Disorder: Molecular Indicators and Relation to Clinical Symptoms

Anna Boyajyan, Gohar Mkrtchyan,
Lilit Hovhannisyan and Diana Avetyan

Additional information is available at the end of the chapter

1. Introduction

Posttraumatic stress disorder (PTSD) (ICD-10 codes: F43.1, F62.0; DSM-IV-TR code: 309.81) [1, 2] is a complex severe and chronic psychiatric illness influenced by environmental and genetic factors [3-10]. PTSD is an anxiety disorder developed in a person experiencing, witnessing, or learning about an extreme physically or psychologically distressing event, associated with unprecedented violence [11, 12]. Traumatic events that can trigger PTSD include massacres, mass murder scenes, international, civil, political, ethnic and religious wars, genocides, natural and man-made disasters, criminal assaults, serious accidents, terrorist attacks, incarceration, trafficking, rape and other types of sexual assaults [12-17], life threatening illness and the sudden death of a loved one, serious medical illness, injury, surgery, hostage, kidnapping, difficult labors, etc [18-20]. Individuals who experience a trauma of this nature may develop symptoms that fall into three distinct clusters: re-experiencing phenomenon; avoidance and numbing; and autonomic hyperarousal. Symptoms usually begin within the first 3 months after the traumatic event and last for many years, although there may be a delay of months, or even years, before symptoms appear. PTSD patients are characterized by severe emotional state, sharp reduction in adaptive and information receiving abilities. They usually remain out of society, become drug addicted, alcoholic and often commit suicide [21-24]. Degrees of risk to develop PTSD from different traumatic events are presented in table 1.

It was shown that 37% of Cambodian refugees, 86% of women refugees in Kabul and Pakistan and 75% of Bosnian refugee women suffer from PTSD. In USA 60% of female rape survivors and 35% of UK adult rape victims are affected by PTSD. Similar to adults, some children, who witness or experience traumatic events, develop PTSD. Thus, in the USA 90-100% of children, who witness a parental homicide or sexual assault, develop PTSD, and in the UK 50% of sexually abused children are affected by this disorder [25-27].

Equally as staggering are statistics, which monitor the incidence of PTSD among combat veterans. Here, 30% of the American Vietnam veterans and 56% of Australia's Vietnam War veterans, 10% of Desert Storm veterans, 31% of Australia's Gulf War veterans, 6-11% of Afghanistan veterans and 12-20% of Iraq veterans in the US suffer from PTSD [25-28].

Statistical data also demonstrates that women are more than twice as likely to develop PTSD as men. Available data suggests that about 8% of men and 20% of women go on to develop PTSD [26, 29-31]. Is was also shown that PTSD is most often developed in representatives of national minorities, people surviving stressful events at list once in their life, as well as in people with low level of education, mental problems, having mentally ill family member or experiencing lack of support from their family members or friends [26, 29-31]. Currently, for about 7-8% of the USA population, 2-3% of the UK population, 6.4% of Australians and 3% of Cambodians suffer from PTSD [26-28].

Traumatic event	Degree of risk, %
Rape	49.0
Other types of sexual violence	23.7
Physical violence, severe beating	31.9
Accident and/or serious injuries	16.8-20.0
Stabbing, shooting	15.4
Sudden death of a family member or friend	14.3
Child's life-threatening illness	10.4
Murder, death or serious injury witness	7.3
Natural disasters - hurricane - tsunami - earthquake (adults/youths)	2.0-3.8 30.0-50.0 32.0-60.0 / 26.0-95.0
Man-made disasters	29.0
Terrorist attacks	28.0

Table 1. Risk for developing PTSD depending on traumatic event [25-27]

In Armenia PTSD is quite common as well, and is basically found among the descendants of Armenian Genocide victims, including current generation, combatants, refugees and victims of earthquake [32-40]. Thus, according to Goenjian et al, 73% among 1988 Spitak Earthquake survivors developed PTSD 4.5 years after the disaster [36]. In general, 10% of the world population is suffering from PTSD, and 70% is under the risk of developing PTSD [26-28].

Patients with PTSD have a reduced quality of life, an increased number of suicides and hospitalizations, high frequency of depressions, alcohol and drug abuse; social, family life and work become impossible.

Molecular mechanisms of generation and development of PTSD and their relation to the clinical psychopathologic criteria of this disorder are not clear yet. The lack of knowledge in this field significantly limits the development of effective therapeutic approaches for treatment of PTSD-affected subjects and prevention of further complications.

2. Neuroendocrine alterations in PTSD

PTSD is characterized by the central and autonomic nervous systems hyperarousal that is caused by functional changes in the limbic system, which is located between the brainstem and the cerebral cortex and coordinates their activities. This part of the brain regulates survival behaviors and emotional expression, being primarily concerned with tasks of survival such as eating, sexual reproduction and the instinctive defenses of fight and flight. It also plays a central role in memory processing. The hippocampus and amygdala, parts of the limbic system, regulate learning, memory, and emotion. The amygdala is important for the regulation of emotional memories, particularly for fear causing memories. It has been proven that amygdala is activated in the extreme situations. The hippocampus, on the contrary, is suppressed in these conditions. It has been shown that PTSD is characterized by functional hyperactivity of the amygdala and hypoactivity of the hippocampus [41-43].

A number of data suggests that alterations in the hypothalamic-pituitary-adrenal (HPA) axis and sympathoadrenal system (SAS) play a leading role in PTSD pathogenesis [13, 14, 44]. Thus, PTSD, as compared to norm, is characterized by low cortisol levels in plasma and saliva [45], whereas elevated levels of dehydroepiandrosterone (DHEA) and DHEA-sulfate are detected in this disorder [44-46]. Moreover, increased levels of corticotrophin realizing hormone positively correlated with the high levels of cortisol in cerebrospinal fluid of PTSD patients were observed [47]. Also, PTSD is characterized by increased glucocorticoid receptor sensitivity [48]. An increased levels of noradrenaline, neurotransmitter of central and peripheral sympathetic (adrenergic) nervous system, were detected in the cerebrospinal fluid of PTSD patients [49]. Noradrenaline is considered as one of the important mediators of central and peripheral autonomic stress response and has an important role in the regulation process of emotional memory [50]. It was also shown that high levels of noradrenalinefof the PTSD of the PTSD in urine positively correlate with the symptoms of PTSD [51]. In addition, the increased levels of dopamine, another mediator of the sympathetic nervous system and precursor of noradrenaline, were found in the blood and body fluids of PTSD-affected subjects [51-53].

There are several data indicating assumption that functional abnormalities in neuroendocrine system detected in PTSD patients are conditioned by hereditary factors [54]. Thus, as it follows from table 2, PTSD is associated with the genetic mutations in a number of genes encoding neurotransmitters and hormones, their biosynthesis enzymes, receptors and transporters. Interestingly, 6 of the candidate genes for PTSD showed in the table 1 belong to the dopamine system. A positive association between the risk for development PTSD and TaqIA polymorphism of the dopamine D2 receptor gene was found [55]. Also, positive association was revealed between tandem repeat polymorphism of dopamine transporter gene and PTSD [56] as well as between dopamine D4 transporter gene long allele and severity of PTSD symptoms [57].

The γ-3 subunit of γ-aminobutyric acid, another mediator of nervous system, has also been studied in PSTD patients. Patients heterozygous for this gene have a higher probability of developing somatic symptoms of PTSD, sleeping disturbances, fair and depression than homozygous patients [58]. The studies of serotonin transporter gene showed that PTSD patients carrying one or two short alleles of this gene have a higher level of depression and suicide compared to carriers of long allele, which has more transcriptional power [59, 60]. The association of the serotonin transporter repeat polymorphism with PTSD was also described [61-63]. Interestingly, recent study of 200 individuals from 12 multigenerational families survived 1998 Spitak earthquake in Armenia demonstrated that PTSD is developing in those individuals, who carry mutations of tryptophan hydroxylase 1 and 2, the rate-limiting enzyme of serotonin biosynthesis [64].

Candidate gene	Chromosomal mapping	Source
Dopamine D2 receptor	11q23	[22, 55, 65]
Dopamine D4 receptor	11p15.5	[57]
Dopamine transporter type 1	5p15.3	[56, 66]
Serotonin transporter	17q11	[10, 60, 63, 67- 71]
Serotonin type-2A receptor	13q14-q21	[68]
Brain-derived neurotrophic factor	11p13	[72]
Neuropeptide Y	7p15.1	[73]
Glucocorticoid receptor	5q31.3	[74]
Dopamine beta-hydroxylase	9q34	[75]
Cannabinoid receptor	6q14-q15	[76]
γ-aminobutyric acid receptor (subunit α-2)	4p12	[77]
Catechol-O-methyltransferase	22q11	[78]
Tryptophan hydroxylase 1 Tryptophan hydroxylase 2	11p15.3-p.14 12q21.1	[64]

Table 2. PTSD-related changes in the neuroendocrine system

3. Immune system alterations in PTSD

Promising studies suggest the involvement of alterations in the immune status [48, 79-86], particularly low-grade inflammatory reactions, in the pathogenesis of PTSD [87-97]. Thus, PTSD patients are characterized by hyperactivation of lymphocytes [80] and increased levels of lipopolysaccharide (LPS)-stimulated expression of interleukin (IL)-6, tumor necrosis factor (TNF)-α, and interferon (IFN)-γ in immunocompetent cells [81, 82]. Segman et al detected over-expression of immune response-related genes in monocytes of PTSD-affected subjects [85]. Also, in chronic PTSD patients, as compared to norm, a decreased number of T-killer cells ($CD8^+$) [98, 99] and an increase number of T-helper cells ($CD4^+$) [98, 100] has been shown, whereas in PTSD patients immediately after a traumatic event a decreased number of T-helper cells was detected [99]. A number of experimental data indicates that natural killer cells' cytotoxicity in PTSD is lower than in norm [97, 99, 101-104], while the total number or these cells, as well as a number of $CD16^+$ and $CD56^+$ cells in their total population is higher than in norm [99, 104]. At the same time some studies show that natural killer cells' cytotoxicity in PTSD patients is higher than in healthy subjects [105, 106]. The analysis of the above mentioned data revealed altered cell-mediated immunity in PTSD patients and demonstrates that depending on traumatic event, duration and stage of the illness, these alterations may be either under- or over-represented [97, 107].

3.1. Cytokine network in PTSD

A number of studies have demonstrated changes in a functional state of cytokines and their receptors, important mediators and regulators of the immune response in PTSD-affected subjects. Here the increased blood levels of proinflammatory cytokines (e.g. IL-1β, IL-6, TNF-α, INF-γ) and decreased levels of anti-inflammatory cytokines (e.g. IL-4) are detected in chronic PTSD patients indicating the involvement of low-grade systemic inflammatory reactions in PTSD pathogenesis (table 3).

In our own study the levels of proinflammatory and chemotactic cytokines IL-1β, IL-6, TNF-α, IL-8 and MCP-1 in the blood serum of chronic PTSD patients (combat veterans) and age- and sex-matched healthy subjects (HS; a control group) were determined using enzyme-linked immunosorbent assay (ELISA). Assessment of possible correlation of the above mentioned parameters with each other and with the expression of PTSD clinical symptoms was also performed. The latest were evaluated using Structured Clinical Interview for the DSM-IV Axis I Disorders (SCID PTSD module) [112] and Clinician-Administered PTSD Scale (CAPS) [113]. In particular, we assessed correlation between the levels of cytokines and the degree of expression of such PTSD clinical symptoms as persistent re-experiencing of the traumatic event (B cluster), persistent avoidance of stimuli associated with the trauma and emotional numbing (C cluster); persistent symptoms of increasing arousal (D cluster) [2]. In table 4 brief descriptions of the study groups is given. Table 5 demonstrates the individual symptom clusters (B, C, and D criteria), and total CAPS scores of PTSD-affected subjects involved in our study.

Chronic PTSD patients: group description	Changes in the blood levels of cytokines as compared to norm*	Source
Accidents survivors (n=13)	↑IL-1β, ↑IL-6, ↑TNF-α	[89]
Accident survivors (n=86)	↑IL-1β	[46]
Accidents survivors (n=14)	↑IL-1β, ↑TNF-α, ↓IL-4	[93]
Bosnian refugees (n=12)	↑IL-6	[108]
Combat veterans (n=19)	↑IL-1β, ↑IL-6, ↑TNF-α	[87]
Combat veterans (n=11)	↑IL-6, ↑TNF-α	[91]
Individuals abused in childhood (n=30)	↑INF-γ	[109]
Individuals abused in childhood (n=177)	↑TNF-α , ↓IL-4	[110]
Individuals exposed to different traumatic events (n=60)	↓IL-4	[97]
Individuals exposed to intimate partner violence (n=62)	↑IL-6, ↑TNF-α, ↑INF-γ	[111]

* - ↑ - above the norm; ↓ - below the norm.

Table 3. Changes in the blood levels of some cytokines in chronic PTSD patients

Data statistics include nonparametric Mann-Whitney U-test and correlation analysis with calculation of Spearman's rank correlation coefficient (Rs). Parts of this study have been published [114, 115].

The results obtained indicated that PTSD, as compared to norm, is characterized by increased levels of the mentioned above cytokines (Table 6), which is consistent with reports by other research groups (Table 3) [46, 87, 89, 91, 93, 108, 110, 111].

A significant correlation between the levels of IL-1β and IL-6 (Rs=0.45; p<0.003), as well as between IL-1β and MCP-1 (Rs=0.3; p<0.03) in PTSD patients was revealed, whereas no significant correlation between the levels of cytokines was observed in control group. Also, a significant positive correlation of IL-1β and IL-6 blood levels with PTSD symptoms within B, C and D criteria (CAPS scores) was detected. Thus, levels of IL-1β positively correlated with B frequency (Rs=0.004, p=0.007), C frequency, intensity, and frequency + intensity (Rs=0.4, p=0.009; Rs=0.30, p=0.035, r=0.36, p<0.02, respectively), frequency of B, C and D (Rs =0.37, p<0.02), total intensity of B, C and D (Rs=0.3, p<0.048) and total frequency + intensity of B, C and D (Rs=0.3, p<0.03). Blood levels of IL-6 positively correlated with cluster B frequency (Rs=0.3, p=0.048).

Our data provides further evidence on the association of chronic inflammation with PTSD and clearly demonstrates the interrelation between the expression of PTSD symptoms and inflammatory reactions. Alterations in the immune response in PTSD accompanied by low-grade systemic inflammation aggravate disease course and severity and contribute to development of complications. Thus, PTSD is often associated with autoimmune and inflammatory disorders such as rheumatoid arthritis, psoriasis and inflammatory bowel disease. Patients with PTSD are at a higher risk for diabetes mellitus and cardiovascular diseases (atherosclerosis, myocardial infarction) [116-123]. It is interesting that in peridontitis patients with PTSD higher expression of inflammatory processes was obtained than in those peridontitis patients, who were not affected by PTSD [88].

Study group	PTSD	HS
Total number (male/female)	120 (116/4)	80 (76/4)
Mean age (M±SD)	42 ± 11.3	39 ± 9.1
[Cortisol]* (M±SD), ng/ml	124 ± 47	145 ± 55
[DHEA]* (M±SD), ng/ml	13 ± 7	10 ± 5
[DHEA-sulfate]* (M±SD), μg/ml	1.8 ± 0.9	1.0 ± 0.5

* - measured in the blood serum

Table 4. Brief description of the study groups

Symptom clusters	Parameters	PTSD patients scores
B cluster	Frequency (0-20)	11.8±3.98
	Intensity (0-20)	11.6±3.46
	Frequency + Intensity (0-40)	23.4±7.02
C cluster	Frequency (0-28)	16.4±5.10
	Intensity (0-28)	14.8±4.96
	Frequency + Intensity (0-56)	31.2±9.85
D cluster	Frequency (0-20)	13.5±3.07
	Intensity (0-20)	12.2±2.52
	Frequency + Intensity (0-40)	25.7±5.30
B+C+D (Total)	Frequency (0-68)	41.7±9.85
	Intensity (0-68)	38.6±9.18
	Frequency + Intensity (0-136)	80.3±18.50

Table 5. The individual symptom clusters (B, C, and D criteria), total and overall CAPS scores (M±SD) of PTSD-affected subjects (Score ranges are indicated in parenthesis)

Study group	Cytokine	Level (M ± SD), pg/ml	P =
PTSD	IL-1β	8.2 ± 1.0	0.002
HS		5.1 ± 0.7	
PTSD	IL-6	19.0 ± 2.5	0.025
HS		16.0 ± 2.3	
PTSD	TNF-α	12.0 ± 1.6	0.049
HS		10.8 ± 1.4	
PTSD	IL-8	11.5 ± 1.5	0.022
HS		10.1 ± 1.3	
PTSD	MCP-1	223.3 ± 30.6	0.030
HS		187.2 ± 25.5	

Table 6. Comparative analysis of the blood serum levels of proinflammatory and chemotactic cytokines in patients with PTSD and HS

The pathological mechanisms of the development of inflammatory reactions in PTSD are not clear. However, it is obvious that neuroendocrine and immune impairments in PTSD are interrelated. It is well-established fact that the immune system functional activity is regulated by neurotransmitters and hormones, particularly those related to HPA axis and SAS. On the other hand, immune system mediators and their receptors on the immunocompetent cells may regulate the neuroendocrine system. In normal physiological conditions the immune, endocrine and nervous systems maintain homeostasis by controlling each other, thus developing adequate stress response [79, 124]. Changes in neuro-endocrine-immune interactions (influenced by either environmental or genetic factors) may result to abnormal response to stress and generation of PTSD. On the other hand, the action of cytokines, mediators of inflammation, is tightly coupled with physiological and pathophysiological reactions of the organism, and their important role is to coordinate the efforts of the immune, endocrine and nervous systems during the stress response [125-128]. This may represent one of the possible mechanisms responsible for increased cytokines levels and development of chronic inflammatory reactions in PTSD, the disease characterized by neuroimmune and endocrine alterations [82, 86, 129]. It connection with this it has to be also mentioned that a number of recent clinical and experimental data suggests the implication of low-grade systemic inflammatory reactions accompanied by increase in cytokines levels in pathogenesis of many psychiatric disorders [130-132].

3.2. The complement system in PTSD

The complement system is major effector of the immune response, which acts on the interface of innate and adaptive immunity, and is a key component and trigger of many immunoregulatory mechanisms. Activation of the complement generates opsonins, anaphylatoxins, and chemotaxins, mediators of inflammation and apoptosis (Figure 1)

[133-135]. Changes in the functional activity of the complement cascade contribute to the pathology of many human diseases [136-138], including mental disorders [139-144], and are also detected during physiological stress [145-146]. The alterations in the complement cascade have been considered as indicator of the implication of inflammatory component in disease etiology, pathogenesis and/or progression [136-138].

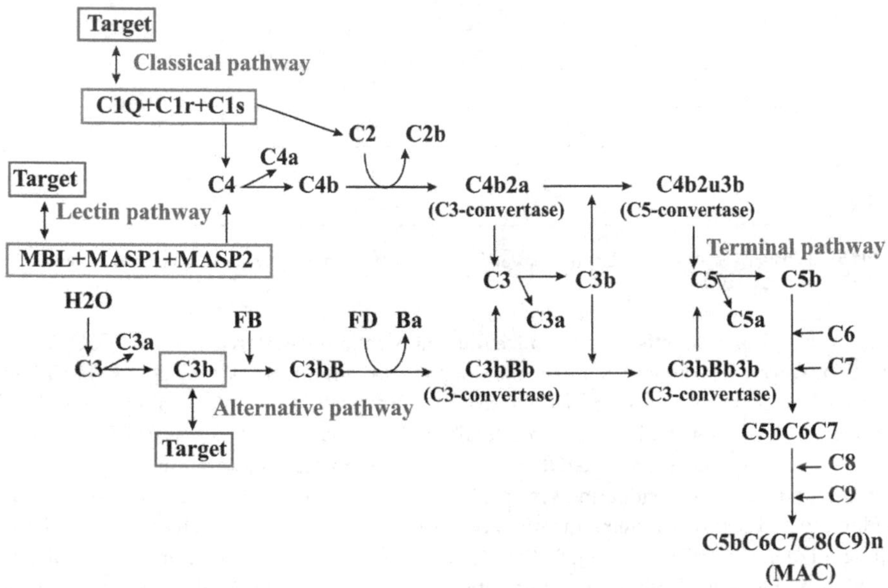

Figure 1. Complement activation pathways; C1Q, C1r, C1s – subunits of the complement C1 component; MBL - mannan-binding lectin; MASP1 - MBL-associated serine peptidase 1; MASP2 - MBL-associated serine peptidase 2; FD - factor D; FB - factor B; MAC – membrane attack complex.

The complement system with its central position in innate and adaptive immunity mediates a variety of effector functions. It consists of more than 30 circulating proteins, cell surface receptor and regulator proteins. It is a complex cascade involving proteolytic cleavage of serum glycoproteins often activated by cell receptors. This cascade ultimately results in induction of the antibody responses, inflammation, phagocyte chemotaxis, and opsonization of apoptotic and necrotic cells, facilitating their recognition, clearance, and lysis. Complement exhibits three activation pathways - classical, alternative, and lectin, initiated via separate mechanisms, and a single terminal pathway that results in a formation of the membrane attack complex (Figure 1) and subsequent cell lysis [133-135]. During the past decades it has become evident that dysfunction of complement contributes to the pathology of many human diseases [136-138], including mental disorders (schizophrenia, Alzheimer's disease, Huntington's and Pick's diseases) [139-142], and is also detected during physiological stress [145-146]. While, as it was already mentioned, PTSD-affected subjects showed a low-grade systemic proinflammatory state, the complement system in PTSD has been never studied before.

In our study we assessed the functional activity of the complement cascade in PTSD by determining total hemolytic activities of its classical and alternative pathways, and hemolytic activities of its individual components, C1, C2, C3, C4, factor B and factor D, in the blood serum of chronic PTSD patients (combat veterans) and HS (tables 4, 5). C1, C2 and C4 are main components of the classical pathway, factor B and factor D are essential components of the alternative pathway, and C3 is the initial point for the alternative pathway and a converge point of all three complement activation pathways, starting up for the terminal pathway (Figure 1) [133-135]. In addition, correlation study between all measured parameters was also performed. Hemolytic activities of the complement classical and alternative pathways (CH50 and AH50, respectively) and of the complement components C1 (C1H50), C2 (C2H50), C3 (C3H50), C4 (C4H50), factor B (fBH50), and factor D (fDH50) in the blood serum of PTSD-affected and healthy subjects were measured by application of the earlier developed methods [147, 148]. Data was analyzed by Student's unpaired two-tailed t-test and Pearson's correlation analysis including calculation of relevant correlation coefficient (r). Parts of this study have been published [149-152].

The results obtained are presented in table 7. According to the results obtained, mean values of serum CH50, C1H50, C2H50 and C4H50 in PTSD patients were significantly 2.1, 1.34, 1.2 and 1.6 times significantly higher than in case of HS ($p<0.05$). On the contrary, mean values of serum C3H50, AH50, fBH50, and fDH50 in PTSD patients were 1.5, 1.7, 1.6, and 2.3 times significantly lower as compared to HS ($p<0.05$). Correlation analysis also demonstrated that in PTSD affected subjects C1H50 is significantly correlated with C2H50 ($r=-0.375$, $p<0.04$), C3H50 is significantly correlated with C1H50, C2H50 and C4H50 and AH50 ($r=0.53$, $p<0.037$; $r=0.72$, $p=0.002$; $r=0.5$, $p=0.05$; $r=0.57$, $p=0.027$, respectively). No significant correlation between the above-mentioned parameters was detected in the HS group ($p>0.05$).

Hemolytic activity, U/ml*	PTSD (M ± SD)	HS (M ± SD)	P =
CH50	375.00 ± 164.40	176.00 ± 88.50	0.0002
C1H50	92.21 ± 52.83	68.80 ± 37.39	0.0400
C2H50	67.60 ± 35.10	58.80 ± 8.80	0.0450
C3H50	37.57 ± 16.26	55.92 ± 28.60	0.0300
C4H50	60.10 ± 28.42	36.64 ± 20.31	0.0300
AH50	52.30 ± 18.17	87.60 ± 9.80	0.0001
fBH50	40.80 ± 14.30	65.2 ± 34.1	0.0200
fBH50	71.70 ± 15.98	163.70 ± 70.58	0.0010

* - one unit (U) of hemolytic activity is defined as an amount of serum that causes a 50% hemolysis of erythrocytes in a reaction mixture.

Table 7. Functional state of the complement system in PTSD patients and HS

The results obtained in our study clearly demonstrated that pathogenesis of PTSD is characterized by complement dysfunction including hyperactivation state of the complement classical pathway and hypoactivation state of the complement alternative pathway. The alternative pathway of complement is activated following spontaneous hydrolysis of the thioester bond of native C3, resulting into binding of factor B, which is cleaved by factor D, generating the efficient alternative pathway C3 convertase C3bBb. Multifunctional complement protein C3 is the initial point of the alternative pathway, and, at the same time, a converge point of all three complement activation pathways, i.e. starting point for the terminal pathway [93, 135, 153]. Hypoactivation state of the alternative pathway together with decreased activity of the complement C3 component, detected in PTSD affected subjects, probably reflects depletion of the C3 component due to its overutilization through the terminal pathway. This suggestion is convenient with correlation data indicating positive correlation between CH50 and C3H50 and absence of any correlation between AH50 and fBH50, and AH50 and fDH50 in PTSD affected subjects. Thus, it is obvious that the alternative pathway in PTSD is suppressed on the initial stage of its activation, and that PTSD is also characterized by overactivated terminal complement pathway. On the other hand, absence of correlation between AH50 and CH50 suggests that alterations in activities of the classical and the alternative complement pathways in PTSD are not interdependent.

As it was mentioned above, alterations in the complement cascade have been considered as indicator of the implication of inflammatory component in disease etiology, pathogenesis and/or progression [136-138]. Our study demonstrates that PTSD is associated with dysfunction of the complement system, and reveals the altered chains of the complement cascade. The results obtained provide further evidence on the involvement of the inflammatory component in pathogenesis of PTSD. Here we hypothesize that neuroendocrine mechanisms related to PTSD modulating the immune function might affect the initial steps in the inflammatory cascade and thus influence alterations in the functional activity of the major mediator of the inflammatory response, the complement system. However, to address molecular mechanisms responsible for the complement dysfunction in PTSD as well as their role in PTSD pathogenesis further studies are needed.

3.3. Immune complexes in PTSD

Formation of immune complexes (IC) is a normal physiological reaction of organism to foreign or autoantigen. IC may interact with both humoral and cellular components of the immune recognition system, activate the complement cascade, and thus affect the immune response on multiple levels [154-156]. In healthy conditions IC are easily eliminating from circulation through complement deposition, followed by their opsonization, phagocytosis, and further processing by proteases [154, 156-158]. In pathologic conditions inappropriate clearance or deposition of IC result in increased levels of IC in circulation. Circulating IC may deposit in endothelial or vascular structures provoking prolonged inflammatory response by permanent activation of the complement cascade through the classical pathway, generation of cytotoxic agents and tissue damage [159-163]. Deposition of IC is a prominent feature of many diseases [162-164] including those characterized by low-grade systemic inflammation, such as schizophrenia [144], diabetes mellitus [165, 166], ischemic and hemorrhagic stroke [167-169].

In our own study we, for the first time, determined total levels of IC as well as the levels of IC containing activation products of the complement system, C1q- and C3d-IC, in the blood serum of chronic PTSD patients (combat veterans) and HS. Brief characteristic of study groups is given in tables 3, 4. Total levels of IC were measured by a previously published spectrophotometric method and expressed in absorbency units at 280 nm (A_{280}) [167]; C1q- and C3d-IC were measured by ELISA. Data was analyzed by Student's unpaired two-tailed t-test and Pearson's correlation analysis including calculation of relevant correlation coefficient (r). Parts of this study have been published [149, 150, 170].

According to the results obtained, PTSD-patients comparing to HS are characterized by significantly increased serum levels of total IC as well as C1q- and C3d-IC. Thus, the mean level of total IC in PTSD patients was 1.5 times higher than in HS (p=0.0055) and the levels of C1q-IC, and C3d-IC were 1.7 (p=0.024) and 1.6 times (p=0.0004), respectively, higher as compared to HS. The results obtained are summarized in table 8.

[IC], (M±SD)	**Study group**		**P =**
	PTSD	**HS**	
[Total IC], A_{280}	0.18 ± 0.1	0.12 ± 0.03	0.0055
[C1q-IC], μg/ml (M±SD)	44.6 ± 37.67	26.28 ± 16.33	0.024
[C3d-IC], μg/ml (M±SD)	29.75 ± 21.91	18.67 ± 8.22	0.0004

Table 8. Serum levels of the total IC, C1q-IC and C3d-IC in PTSD patients and HS

In addition, a significant positive correlation between the levels of C1q- and C3d-IC (r=0.32; p<0.03) was detected in PTSD patients affected subjects. Moreover, in patients with PTSD we also revealed a significant positive correlation between the total levels of IC and hemolytic activity of the classical complement pathway. This finding indicates that increased total levels of IC in circulation may be responsible for hyperactivation of the classical complement cascade detected in PTSD [149-152, 170].

The increased blood levels of C1q-IC in PTSD provide further evidence for this suggestion. C1q-IC contain C1q subunit of the complement protein C1, and binding of IC to C1q initiates activation of the classical complement cascade (Figure 1) [133-135].

C3d-IC contain activation cleavage products of the complement C3 protein, opsonins C3b, iC3b and C3dg. These entire products contain "d"-terminal fragment of the C3 polypeptide chain. In healthy conditions C3d-IC are eliminated from the blood through interaction with the complement receptors on monocytes, neutrophils and erythrocytes. Monocytes and neutrophils subject C3d-IC to phagocytosis, and erythrocytes transfer them to liver and spleen for further phagocytosis by macrophages. Increased blood levels of C3d-IC suggest about alterations in mechanisms responsible for their recognition and clearance by the above mentioned cells. High levels of C3d-IC result in hyper-production of antibodies, because binding of C3d-IC to type-2 complement receptors (CR2) on the surface of B-lymphocytes induces the production of immunoglobulins by these cells [154, 156-158]. Therefore, our results indicate that PTSD is characterized by altered mechanisms of IC recognition and clearance, which may be responsible for the increased classical pathway functional activity, chronic activation of the immune system and systemic inflammation.

3.4. Interrelation between inflammatory response, apoptosis and synaptic plasticity in PTSD

As it was already mentioned, the molecular pathomechanisms responsible for development of inflammatory reactions in PTSD are yet unclear, which limits the progress in development of the efficient measures of PTSD rehabilitation therapy and prevention of its complications. On the other hand, it is known that apoptosis plays an important role in down-regulation of the inflammatory response by reducing the lifespan of activated immunocompetent cells [171-173]. Therefore, we proposed that one of the factors contributing to PTSD-associated inflammation may be apoptotic dysfunction as it was observed in case of other disorders like familial Mediterranean fever [174], inflammatory bowel disease [175], systemic inflammatory response syndrome [176], pulmonary hemorrhage or endotoxemia [177], etc.

On the third though, apoptosis is considered as the important regulator of synaptic plasticity. Apoptotic alterations have a significant input in synaptic dysfunction and lead to changes in structural and functional integrity of neuronal circuits [178-180]. Therefore, apoptosis may be also responsible for altered synaptic plasticity in PTSD [181] resulting in cognitive impairments and development of depressions in PTSD affected subjects [182-184].

To check our hypotheses, in the blood serum of patients with PTSD, in comparison to HS the levels of marker proteins for apoptosis and synaptic plasticity, annexin-A5 [185] and complexin-2 [186], respectively, and the inflammatory marker, TNF-α, were determined by ELISA. The analysis of correlation between these parameters was performed. Brief characteristic of study groups is given in tables 4, 5. Data statistics include nonparametric Mann-Whitney U-test and correlation analysis with calculation of Spearman's rank correlation coefficient (Rs). The results presented below have not been published yet.

According to the results obtained, the levels of both annexin-A5 and complexin-2 in PTSD patients were significantly 2.34 ($p=0.0001$) and 1.21 ($p=0.03$) times, respectively, lower than in case of HS (table 9). In addition, a significant positive correlation between the levels of annexin-A5 and complexin-2 ($Rs=0.38$, $p=0.045$), on the one hand, and a significant negative correlation between the levels of annexin-A5 and the increased levels of TNF-α ($Rs= -0.35$, $p=0.047$), on the other hand, were detected in PTSD.

No statistical significant correlation was observed between these parameters in case of HS.

Study group	[Annexin-A5], ng/ml	P =	[Complexin-2], pg/ml	P =
PTSD	0.82 ± 0.70	0.0001	121.5 ± 41.20	0.03
HS	1.92 ± 1.05		146.9 ± 56.64	

Table 9. The levels of annexin A5 and complexin-2 (M ± SD) in PTSD patients and HS

Our results demonstrated that PTSD is characterized by the decreased blood levels of the apoptotic marker circulating annexin A5 indicating association of apoptosis hypofunction with this disorder.

On the base of the results obtained we suggest that PTSD is characterized by low rate of apoptosis associated with the defects in synaptic plasticity and that anomalous apoptosis may also represent one of the factors responsible for development of PTSD-associated chronic inflammation. This suggestion is confirmed by recent findings indicating the increased levels of leukocytes in the blood of chronic PTSD patients [48, 93, 94].

4. Conclusion

The results presented in this chapter provide evidence on implication of altered immune response, particularly low-grade systemic inflammation, in pathogenesis of PTSD.

In particular, we demonstrated that chronic PTSD is characterized by increased blood levels of proinflammatory and chemotactic cytokines, IL-1β, IL-6, TNF-α and MCP-1, IL-8, respectively. Here, the increased levels of IL-1β and IL-6 positively correlate with the degree of expression of clinically significant symptoms of this disease, which indicate that these cytokines may be considered as new therapeutic targets for PTSD treatment. In addition, we demonstrated that chronic PTSD is characterized by altered mechanisms of IC recognition and clearance resulting in the increased levels of total IC, as well as C1q-IC and C3d-IC in circulation. Furthermore, our results showed that chronic PTSD is characterized by alterations in functional activity of the complement pathways including hyperactivation state of the classical and terminal pathways, hypoactivation state of the alternative pathway and deficiency of the C3 complement protein. Here, the data obtained suggests that hyperactivation of the classical complement pathway is induced by the increased levels of IC, particularly C1q-IC, in circulation. Regarding the alternative pathway, our results clearly demonstrated that it is suppressed at the initial stage of activation and that decreased activity of this pathway in PTSD is stipulated by decreased activities of its components, factor B and factor D, and deficiency of the protein C3, a key component of the complement cascade.

In summery, we concluded that changes in functional activities of the proinflammatory and chemotactic cytokines and complement cascade, as well as disturbances in the IC recognition and clearance processes are implicated in pathogenesis of chronic PTSD.

Another important conclusion that can be drawn from the results of our study is that pathogenesis of chronic PTSD is characterized by low rate of apoptosis associated with the defects in synaptic plasticity, and that anomalous apoptosis may represent one of the factors responsible for development of PTSD-associated chronic inflammation.

Author details

Anna Boyajyan, Gohar Mkrtchyan, Lilit Hovhannisyan and Diana Avetyan

*Address all correspondence to: aboyajyan@sci.am

Institute of Molecular Biology, National Academy of Sciences, Yerevan, Republic of Armenia

References

[1] ICD-10. International statistical classification of diseases and related health problems (Edition: 10). Geneva: World Health Organization; 1992.

[2] DSM-IV-TR. Diagnostic and statistical manual of mental disorders by the American Psychiatric Association (edition 4, text revised). USA: Amer. Psych. Pub; 2000.

[3] Segman RH, Shalev AY. Genetics of posttraumatic stress disorder. CNS Spectr 2003;8(9): 693-698.

[4] Eley TC, Sugden K, Corsico A, Gregory AM, Sham P. Gene-environment interaction analysis of serotonin system markers with adolescent depression. Mol Psychiatry 2004;9(10): 908-915.

[5] Grabe HJ, Lange M, Wolff B, Völzke H, Lucht M. Mental and physical distress is modulated by a polymorphism in the 5-HT transporter gene interacting with social stressors and chronic disease burden. Mol Psychiatry 2005;10(2): 220-224.

[6] Koenen KC. Genetics of posttraumatic stress disorder: review and recommendations for future studies. J Trauma Stress 2007;20: 737-750.

[7] Binder EB, Bradley RG, Liu W, Epstein MP, Deveau TC, Mercer KB, Tang Y, Gillespie CF, Heim CM, Nemeroff CB, Schwartz AC, Cubells JF, Ressler KJ. Association of FKBP5 polymorphisms and childhood abuse with risk of posttraumatic stress disorder symptoms in adults. JAMA 2008; 299(11) 1291-1305.

[8] Amstadter AB, Nugent NR, Koenen KC. Genetics of PTSD: fear conditioning as a model for future research. Psych Ann 2009;39: 358-367.

[9] Koenen KC, Aiello AE, Bakshis E, Amstadter AB, Ruggiero KJ, Acierno R, Kilpatrick DG, Gelernter J, Galea S. Modification of the association between serotonin transporter genotype and risk of posttraumatic stress disorder in adults by county-level social environment. Am J Epidemiol 2009;169: 704-711.

[10] Mellman TA, Alim T, Brown DD, Gorodetsky E, Buzas B, Lawson WB, Goldman D, Charney DS. Serotonin polymorphisms and posttraumatic stress disorder in a trauma exposed African American population. Depress Anxiety 2009;26: 993-997.

[11] Shalev AY, Peri T, Orr SP, Bonne O, Pitman RK. Auditory startle responses in help seeking trauma survivors. Psych Res 1997;69: 1-7.

[12] Dietrich AM. As the pendulum swings: The etiology of PTSD, complex PTSD, and revictimization. Traumatology 2000;6: 41-59.

[13] Yehuda R, Giller EL, Levengood RA, Southwick SM, Siever LJ. Hypotalamic-pituitary-adrenal functioning in post-traumatic stress disorder: expanding the concept of the stress response specrtum. Neurobiologial and clinical consequences of stress: from normal adaptation to post-traumatic stress disorder. Hagerstown. MD: Lippincott-Raven; 1991. p351-366.

[14] Yehuda R. Biology of posttraumatic stress disorder. J Clin Psychiatry 2001;62(17): 41-46.

[15] Roth S, Newman E, Pelcovitzl D. Complex PTSD in victims exposed to sexual and physical abuse: results from the DSM-IV field trial for posttraumatic stress disorder. J Trauma Stress 1997;10(4): 539-545.

[16] Connor MD, Butterfield MI. Post-traumatic stress disorder. FOCUS 2003;1(3): 247-262.

[17] Kinchin D. Post traumatic stress disorder: the invisible injury. UK: Success Unlimited; 2005.

[18] Beck CT. Birth trauma: in the eye of the beholder. Nurs Res 2004;53(1): 28-35.

[19] Beck CT. Post-traumatic stress disorder due to childbirth: the aftermath. Nurs Res 2004;53(4): 216-224.

[20] Aldecoa C, Pico S, Rico J, Vazquez B, Gomez L, Garcia-Bernardo C, Gomez-Herreras J. Post-traumatic stress disorder after surgical ICU admission. Crit Care 2010;14(1): 441.

[21] Amir M, Kaplan Z, Efroni R, Kotler M. Suicide risk and coping styles in post-traumatic stress disorder patients. Psychother Psychosom 1999;68(2): 76-81.

[22] Young RM, Lawford BR, Noble EP, Kann B, Wilkie A, Ritchie T, Arnold L, Shadforth S. Harmful drinking in military veterans with post-traumatic stress disorder: association with the D2 dopamine receptor A1 allele. Alcohol 2002;37(5): 451-456.

[23] Ben-Ya'acov Y, Amir M. Posttraumatic symptoms and suicide risk. Person Indiv Diff 2004;36: 1257-1264.

[24] Tull M. The Connection Between PTSD and alcohol and drug use. Posttraumatic stress. New York: About.com 2008. http://ptsd.about.com/od/relatedconditions/a/drugalcohol.htm.

[25] Picking up the peaces (n.d.). Raising awareness about PTSD. 2012. http://pickingupthepeaces.org.au/post-traumatic-stress-disorder-statistics/ (accessed 25 February 2012).

[26] PTSD alliance (n.d.). About PTSD: statistics. 2012. www.ptsdalliance.org/about_what.html. (accessed 25 February 2012).

[27] HMForces.co.uk (n.d.). Post traumatic stress disorder - helping family with PTSD. 2012. http://www.hmforces.co.uk/education/articles/593-post-traumatic-stress-disorder-helping-family-with-ptsd. (accessed 25 February 2012).

[28] Creamer MC, Burgess P, McFarlane AC. Post-traumatic stress disorder: findings from the Australian National Survey of Mental Health and Well-being. Psychol Med 2001;31(7): 1237-1247.

[29] Helzer JE, Robins LN, McEvoy L. Post-traumatic stress disorder in the general population. Findings of the epidemiologic catchment area survey. N Engl J Med 1987;317(26): 1630-1634.

[30] Breslau N. The epidemiology of posttraumatic stress disorder: what is the extent of the problem? J Clin Psychiatry 2001;62(17): 16-22.

[31] Breslau N. Epidemiologic studies of trauma, posttraumatic stress disorder, and other psychiatric disorders. Can J Psychiatry 2002;47(10): 923-929.

[32] Goenjian AK. A mental health relief programme in Armenia after the 1988 earthquake. Br J Psychiatry 1993;163: 230-239.

[33] Bakunts AG. Mental disorders among Armenian volunteers fighting in Karabakh. Bekhterev Rev Psychiatr Med Psychol 1994(2): 77-79.

[34] Goenjian AK, Najarian LM, Pynoos RS, Steinberg AM, Manoukian G, Tavosian A, Fairbanks LA. Posttraumatic stress disorder in elderly and younger adults after the 1988 earthquake in Armenia. Am J Psychiatry 1994;151: 895-901.

[35] Azarian A, Skriptchenko-Gregorian V. Children in natural disasters: an experience of the 1988 earthquake in Armenia. US: American Academy of Experts in Traumatic Stress Inc; 1998. http://www.aaets.org/article38.htm

[36] Goenjian AK, Steinberg AM, Najarian LM, Fairbanks LA, Tashjian M, Pynoos RS. Prospective study of posttraumatic stress, anxiety, and depressive reactions after earthquake and political violence. Am J Psychiatry 2000;157: 911-916.

[37] Goenjian AK, Pynoos RS, Steinberg AM, Endres D, Abraham K, Geffner ME, Fairbanks LA. Hypothalamic-pituitary-adrenal activity among Armenian adolescents with PTSD symptoms. J Traumatic Stress 2003;16(4): 319-323.

[38] Sukiasyan SH, Tadevosyan AS, Jeshmaridian SS, Manasyan NG. Stress and post stress disorders: personality and society. Yerevan: Asoghik Publishing House; 2003.

[39] Sukiasyan SH, Tadevosyan MJ. Posttraumatic stress disorder: medical and social - psychological problem in Armenia. Russ J Psychiatry 2010;5: 59-69.

[40] Karenian H, Livaditis M, Karenian S, Zafiriadis K, Bochtsou V, Xenitidis K. Collective trauma transmission and traumatic reactions among descendants of Armenian refugees. Int J Soc Psychiatry 2011;57(4): 327-337.

[41] Sapolsky RM. Atrophy of the hippocampus in posttraumatic stress disorder: how and when? Hippocampus 2001;11: 90-91.

[42] Shin LM, Shin PS, Heckers S, Krangel TS, Mackli ML, Orr SP. Hippocampal function in posttraumatic stress disorder. Hippocampus 2004;14: 292-300.

[43] Karl A, Schaefer M, Malta LS, Dorfel D, Rohleder N, Werner A. A meta-analysis of structural brain abnormalities in PTSD. Neurosci Biobehav Rev 2006;30(7): 1004-1031.

[44] Heim C, Ehlert U, Hellhammer DH. The potential role of hypocortisolism in the pathophysiology of stress-related bodily disorders. Psychoneuroendocrinology 2000;25: 1-35.

[45] Gill JM, Vythilingam M, Page GG. Low cortisol, high DHEA, and high levels of stimulated TNF-α, and IL-6 in women with PTSD. J Trauma Stress 2008;21(6): 530-539.

[46] Tucker P, Ruwe WD, Masters B. Neuroimmune and cortisol changes in selective serotonin reuptake inhibitor and placebo treatment of chronic posttraumatic stress disorder. Biol Psychiatry 2004;56: 121-128.

[47] Carpenter LL, Tyrka AR, McDougle CJ, Malison RT, Owens MJ, Nemeroff CB, Price LH. Cerebrospinal fluid corticotropin-releasing factor and perceived early-life stress in depressed patients and healthy control subjects. Neuropsychopharmacology 2004;29(4): 777-784.

[48] De Kloet CS, Vermetten E, Bikker A, Meulman E, Geuze E, Kavelaars A, Westenberg HG, Heijnen CJ. Leukocyte glucocorticoid receptor expression and immunoregulation in veterans with and without post-traumatic stress disorder. Mol Psychiatry 2007;12(5):443-453.

[49] Geracioti TD. Plasma and cerebrospinal fluid interleukin-6 concentrations in posttraumatic stress disorder. Neuroimmunomodulation 2001;9: 209-217.

[50] Heim C, Nemeroff CB. Neurobiology of posttraumatic stress disorder. CNS Spectr 2009;14(1): 13-24.

[51] Yehuda R, Southwick S, Giller EL, Ma X, Mason JW. Urinary catecholamine excretion and severity of PTSD symptoms in Vietnam combat veterans. J Nerv Ment Dis 1992;180(5): 321-325.

[52] Hamner MB, Diamond BI. Elevated plasma dopamine in posttraumatic stress disorder: a preliminary report. Biol Psychiatry 1993;33(4): 304-306.

[53] Glover DA, Powers MB, Bergman L, Smits JAJ, Telch MJ, Stube M. Urinary dopamine and turn bias in traumatized women with and without PTSD symptoms. Behavioural Brain Research 2003;144: 137-141.

[54] Pivac N, Kozarić-Kovačić D. Neurobiology of PTSD. In: Begec S. (ed.) The integration and management of traumatized people after terrorist attack. Amsterdam: IOS Press; 2007. p41-62.

[55] Comings DE, Muhleman D, Gysin R. Dopamine D2 receptor (DRD2) gene and susceptibility to posttraumatic stress disorder: a study and replication. Biol Psychiatry 1996;40: 368-372.

[56] Segman RH, Cooper-Kazaz R, Macciardi F, Goltser T, Halfon Y, Dobroborski T, Shalev AY. Association between the dopamine transporter gene and posttraumatic stress disorder. Mol Psychiatry 2002;7: 903-907.

[57] Dragan WL, Oniszczenko W. The association between dopamine D4 receptor exon III polymorphism and intensity of PTSD symptoms among flood survivors. Anxiety Stress Coping 2009;22: 483-495.

[58] Feusner J, Ritchie T, Lawford B, Young RM, Kann B, Noble EP. GABA(A) receptor beta 3 subunit gene and psychiatric morbidity in a post-traumatic stress disorder population. Psychiatry Res 2001;104(2): 109-117.

[59] Lesch KP, Bengel D, Heils A, Sabol SZ, Greenberg BD, Petri S, Benjamin J, Muller CR, Hamer DH, Murphy DL. Association of anxiety-related traits with a polymorphism in the serotonin transporter gene regulatory region. Science 1996;274(5292): 1527-1531.

[60] Kilpatrick DG, Koenen KC, Ruggiero KJ, Acierno R, Galea S, Resnick HS, Roitzsch J, Boyle J, Gelernter J. The serotonin transporter genotype and social support and moderation of posttraumatic stress disorder and depression in hurricane exposed adults. Am J Psychiatry 2007;164: 1693-1699.

[61] Eley TC, Sugden K, Corsico A, Gregory AM, Sham P. Gene-environment interaction analysis of serotonin system markers with adolescent depression. Mol Psychiatry 2004;9(10): 908-915.

[62] Kendler KS, Kuhn JW, Vittum J, Prescott CA, Riley B. The interaction of stressful life events and a serotonin transporter polymorphism in the prediction of episodes of major depression: a replicatio. Arch Gen Psychiatry 2005;62(5): 529-535.

[63] Grabe HJ, Spitzer C, Schwahn C, Marcinek A, Frahnow A, Barnow S, Lucht M, Freyberger HJ, John U, Wallaschofski H, Völzke H, Rosskopf D. Serotonin transporter gene (SLC6A4) promoter polymorphisms and the susceptibility to posttraumatic stress disorder in the general population. Am J Psychiatry 2009; 166: 926-933.

[64] Goenjian AK, Bailey JN, Walling DP, Steinberg AM, Schmidt D, Dandekar U, NobleEP. Association of TPH1, TPH2, and 5HTTLPR with PTSD and depressive symptoms. J Affect Disord 2012 [Epub ahead of print].

[65] Voisey J, Swagell CD, Hughes IP, Morris CP, Van Daal A, Noble EP, Kann B, Heslop KA, Young RM, Lawford BR. The DRD2 gene 957C > T polymorphism is associated with posttraumatic stress disorder in war veterans. Depress Anxiety 2009;6(1): 28-33.

[66] Drury SS, Theall KP, Keats BJ, Scheeringa M. The role of the dopamine transporter (DAT) in the development of PTSD in preschool children. J Trauma Stress 2009;22: 534-539.

[67] Lee HJ, Lee MS, Kang RH, Kim H, Kim SD, Kee BS, Kim YH, Kim YK, Kim JB, Yeon BK, Oh KS, Oh BH, Yoon JS, Lee C, Jung HY, Chee IS, Paik IH. Influence of the serotonin transporter promoter gene polymorphism on susceptibility to posttraumatic stress disorder. Depress Anxiety 2005;21: 135-139.

[68] Lee H, Kwak S, Paik J, Kang R, Lee M. Association between serotonin 2A receptor gene polymorphism and posttraumatic stress disorder. Psychiatry Investig 2007;4: 104-108.

[69] Thakur GA, Joober R, Brunet A. Development and persistence of posttraumatic stress disorder and the 5-HTTLPR polymorphism. J Trauma Stress 2009;22: 240-243.

[70] Xie P, Kranzler HR, Poling J, Stein MB, Anton RF, Brady K, Weiss RD, Farrer L, Gelernter J. Interactive effect of stressful life events and the serotonin transporter 5-HTTLPR genotype on posttraumatic stress disorder diagnosis in 2 independent populations. Arch Gen Psychiatry 2009;66: 1201-1209.

[71] Sayin A, Kucukyildirim S, Akar T, Bakkaloglu Z, Demircan A, Kurtoglu G, Demirel B, Candansayar S, Mergen H. A prospective study of serotonin transporter gene promoter (5-HTT gene linked polymorphic region) and intron 2 (variable number of tandem repeats) polymorphisms as predictors of trauma response to mild physical injury. DNA Cell Biol 2010;29: 71-77.

[72] Zhang H, Ozbay F, Lappalainen J, Kranzler HR, van Dyck CH, Charney DS, Price LH, Southwick S, Yang BZ, Rasmussen A, Gelernter J. Brain derived neurotrophic factor (BDNF) gene variants and Alzheimer's disease, affective disorders, posttraumatic stress disorder, schizophrenia, and substance dependence. Am J Med Genet B Neuropsychiatr Genet 2006;141: 387-393.

[73] Lappalainen J, Kranzler HR, Malison R, Price LH, Van Dyck C, Rosenheck RA, Cramer J, Southwick S, Charney D, Krystal J, Gelernter J. A functional neuropeptide Y Leu7Pro polymorphism associated with alcohol dependence in a large population sample from the United States. Arch Gen Psychiatry 2002;59: 825-831.

[74] Bachmann AW, Sedgley TL, Jackson RV. Glucocorticoid receptor polymorphisms and post-traumatic stress disorder. Psychoneuroendocrinology 2005;30: 297-306.

[75] Mustapic M, Pivac N, Kozaric-Kovacic D, Dezeljin M, Cubells JF, Mück-Seler D. Dopamine beta-hydroxylase (DBH) activity and -1021C/T polymorphism of DBH gene in combat-related post-traumatic stress disorder. Am J Med Genet Neuropsychiatr Genet 2007;144B(8): 1087-1089.

[76] Lu AT, Ogdie MN, Jarvelin MR, Moilanen IK, Loo SK, McCracken JT, McGough JJ, Yang MH, Peltonen L, Nelson SF, Cantor RM, Smalley SL. Association of the cannabinoid receptor gene (CNR1) with ADHD and posttraumatic stress disorder. Am J Med Gene Neuropsychiatr Genet 2008;147B: 1488-1494.

[77] Nelson EC, Agrawal A, Pergadia ML, Lynskey MT, Todorov AA, Wang JC, Todd RD, Martin NG, Heath AC, Goate AM, Montgomery GW, Madden PA. Association of childhood trauma exposure and GABRA2 polymorphisms with risk of posttraumatic stress disorder in adults. Mol Psychiatry 2009;14: 234-235.

[78] Kolassa IT, Kolassa S, Ertl V, Papassotiropoulos A, De Quervain DJ. The risk of posttraumatic stress disorder after trauma depends on traumatic load and the catechol-o-methyltransferase Val(158)Met polymorphism. Biol Psychiatry 2010;67: 304-308.

[79] Miller AH. Neuroendocrine and immune system interactions in stress and depression. Psychiatr Clin North Am 1998;21: 443-463.

[80] Wilson SN, Van der Kolk B, Burbridge J, Fisler R, Kradin R. Phenotype of blood lymphocytes in PTSD suggests chronic immune activation. Psychosomatics 1999;40(3): 222-225.

[81] Kawamura N, Kim Y, Asukai N. Suppression of cellular immunity in men with a past history of posttraumatic stress disorder. Am J Psych 2001;158: 484-486.

[82] Wong CM. Post-traumatic stress disorder: advances in psychoneuroimmunology. Psychiatr Clin North Am 2002;25(2): 369-383.

[83] Altemus M, Enhanced cellular immune response in women with PTSD related to childhood abuse. Am J Psych 2003;160: 1705-1707.

[84] Everson MP, Kotler S, Blackburn WD. PTSD and immune dysregulation in gulf war veterans. Med. Eval. Programs VA Gulf War Registry. 2005. https://www.gulflink.osd.mil/medical.

[85] Segman RH, Shefi N, Goltser-Dubner T, Friedman N, Kaminski N, Shalev AY. Peripheral blood mononuclear cell gene expression profiles identify emergent posttraumatic stress disorder among trauma survivors. Mol. Psychiatry 2005;10: 500-513.

[86] Altemus M, Dhabhar FS, Yang R. Immune function in PTSD. Ann NY Acad Sci 2006;1071: 167-183.

[87] Spivak B, Shohat B, Mester R, Avraham S, Gil-Ad I, Bleich A, Valevski A, Weizman A. Elevated levels of serum interleukin-1 beta in combat-related posttraumatic stress disorder. Biol Psychiatry 1997;42(5): 345-348.

[88] Aurer A, Aurer-Kozelj J, Stavljenic-Rukavina A, Kalenic S, Ivic-Kardu M, Haban V. Infammatory mediators in saliva of patients with rapidly progressive periodontis during war stress induced incidence increase. Coll Antropol 1999;23: 117-124.

[89] Maes M, Lin AH., Delmeire L, Van Gastel A, Kenis G, De Jongh R, Bosmans E. Elevated serum interleukin-6 (IL-6) and IL-6 receptor concentrations in posttraumatic

stress disorder following accidental man-made traumatic events. Biol Psychiatry 1999;45(7): 833-839.

[90] Miller RJ, Sutherland AG, Hutchinson JD, Alexander DA. C-reactive protein and interleukin 6 receptor in post-traumatic stress disorder: a pilot study. Cytokine 2001;13: 253-255.

[91] Baker DG, Ekhator NN, Kasckow JW, Hill KK, Zoumakis E, Dashevsky BA, Chrousos GP, Geracioti TD. Plasma and cerebrospinal fluid interleukin-6 concentrations in posttraumatic stress disorder. Neuroimmunomodulation 2001;9(4): 209-217.

[92] Wessa M, Rohleder N. Endocrine and inflammatory alterations in post-traumatic stress disorder. Expert Rev Endocrinol Metab 2007;2(1): 91-122.

[93] von Känel R, Hepp U, Kraemer B, Traber R, Keel M, Mica L, Schnyder U. Evidence for low-grade systemic proinflammatory activity in patients with posttraumatic stress disorder. J Psychiatr Res 2007;41(9): 744-752.

[94] Gill JM, Saligan L, Woods S, Page G. PTSD is associated with an excess of inflammatory immune activities. Perspect Psychiatr Care 2009;45(4): 262-277.

[95] Spitzer C, Barnow S, Völzke H, Wallaschofski H, John U, Freyberger HJ, Löwe B, Grabe HJ. Association of posttraumatic stress disorder with low-grade elevation of C-reactive protein: Evidence from the general population. J Psychiatr Res 2010;44(1): 15-21.

[96] Von Känel R, Begré S, Abbas ChC, Saner H, Gander ML, Schmid JP. Inflammatory biomarkers in patients with posttraumatic stress disorder caused by myocardial infarction and the role of depressive symptoms. Neuroimmunomodulation 2010;17(1): 39-46.

[97] Kawamura N, Kim Y, Asukai N. Suppression of cellular immunity in men with a past history of posttraumatic stress disorder. Am J Psych 2001;158: 484-486.

[98] Glover DA, Steele AC, Stuber ML, Fahey JL. Preliminary evidence for lymphocyte distribution differences at rest and after acute psychological stress in PTSD-symptomatic women. Brain Behav Immun 2005;19(3): 243-251.

[99] Ironson G, Wynings C, Schneiderman N, Baum A, Rodriguez M, Greenwood D, Benight C, Antoni M, LaPerriere A, Huang HS, Klimas N, Fletcher MA. Posttraumatic stress symptoms, intrusive thoughts, loss, and immune function after Hurricane Andrew. Psychosom Med 1997;59(2): 128-141.

[100] Vidović A, Gotovac K, Vilibić M, Sabioncello A, Jovanović T, Rabatić S, Folnegović-Šmalć V, Dekaris D. Repeated assessments of endocrine- and immune-related changes in posttraumatic stress disorder. Neuroimmunomodulation 2011;18(4): 199-211.

[101] Mosnaim AD, Wolf ME, Maturana P, Mosnaim G, Puente J, Kucuk O, Gilman-Sachs A. In vitro studies of natural killer cell activity in post traumatic stress disorder pa-

tients. Response to methionine-enkephalin challenge. Immunopharmacology 1993;25(2): 107-116.

[102] Inoue-Sakurai C, Maruyama S, Morimoto K. Posttraumatic stress and lifestyles are associated with natural killer cell activity in victims of the Hanshin-Awaji earthquake in Japan. Prev Med 2000;31(5): 467-473.

[103] Gotovac K, Vidović A, Vukusić H, Krcmar T, Sabioncello A, Rabatić S, Dekaris D. Natural killer cell cytotoxicity and lymphocyte perforin expression in veterans with posttraumatic stress disorder. Prog Neuropsychopharmacol Biol Psychiatry 2010;34(4): 597-604.

[104] Skarpa I, Rubesa G, Moro L, Manestar D, Petrovecki M, Rukavina D. Changes of cytolytic cells and perforin expression in patients with posttraumatic stress disorder. Croat Med J 2001;42(5): 551-555.

[105] Delahanty DL, Dougall AL, Craig KJ, Jenkins FJ, Baum A. Chronic stress and natural killer cell activity after exposure to traumatic death. Psychosom Med 1997;59(5): 467-476.

[106] Laudenslager ML, Aasal R, Adler L, Berger CL, Montgomery PT, Sandberg E, Wahlberg LJ, Wilkins RT, Zweig L, Reite ML. Elevated cytotoxicity in combat veterans with long-term post-traumatic stress disorder: preliminary observations. Brain Behav Immun 1998;12(1): 74-79.

[107] Boscarino JA, Chang J. Higher abnormal leukocyte and lymphocyte counts 20 years after exposure to severe stress: research and clinical implications. Psychosom Med 1999;61(3): 378-386.

[108] Rohleder N, Joksimovic L, Wolf JM, Kirschbaum C. Hypocortisolism and increased glucocorticoid sensitivity of pro-Inflammatory cytokine production in Bosnian war refugees with posttraumatic stress disorder. Biol Psychiatry 2004;1(55):745-751.

[109] Grassi-Oliveira R, Brietzke E, Pezzi JC, Lopes RP, Teixeira AL, Bauer ME. Increased soluble tumor necrosis factor-alpha receptors in patients with major depressive disorder. Psychiatry Clin Neurosci 2009;63(2):202-208.

[110] Smith AK, Conneely KN, Kilaru V, Mercer KB, Weiss TE, Bradley B, Tang Y, Gillespie CF, Cubells JF, Ressler KJ. Differential immune system DNA methylation and cytokine regulation in post-traumatic stress disorder. Am J Med Genet B Neuropsychiatr Genet 2011;156(6): 700-708.

[111] Woods AB, Page GG, O'Campo P. The mediation effect of posttraumatic stress disorder symptoms on the relationship of intimate partner violence and IFN-gamma levels. Am J Community Psychol 2005;36: 159-175.

[112] First MB, Spitzer RL, Gibbon M, Williams JB. Structured clinical interview for the DSM-IV® axis I disorders (SCID-I), clinician version, user's guide. USA: Am Psych Press Inc; 1997.

[113] Blake DD, Weathers FW, Nagy LM, Kaloupek DG, Gusman FD, Charney DS, Keane TM. The development of a clinician administered PTSD scale. J Trauma Stress 1995;8(1): 75-90.

[114] Hovhannisyan LP, Mkrtchyan GM, Sukiasian SH, Boyajyan AS. Classic and alternative complement cascades in post-traumatic stress disorder. Bull Exper Biol Medic 2009;148(6): 859-861.

[115] Hovhannisyan LP, Mkrtchyan GM, Boyajyan AS, Avetyan DG, Tadevosyan MY, Sukiasyan SH. Inflammatory markers in post-traumatic stress disorder. Cytokines & Inflammation 2012;11(1): 42-45.

[116] Boscarino JA. Diseases among men 20 years after exposure to severe stress: implications for clinical research and medical care. Psychosom Med 1997;59: 605-614.

[117] Boscarino JA, Chang J. Electrocardiogram abnormalities among men with stress-related psychiatric disorders: implications for coronary heart disease and clinical research. Ann Behav Med 1999;21: 227-234.

[118] Weisberg RB, Bruce SE, Machan JT, Kessler RC, Culpepper L, Keller MB. Nonpsychiatric illness among primary care patieints with trauma histories and posttraumatic stress disorder. Psychiatr Serv 2002;53: 848-854.

[119] Kimerling R. An investigation of sex differences in non-psychiatric morbidity associated with posttraumatic stress disorder. J Am Med Womens Assoc 2004;59: 43-47.

[120] Boscarino JA. Posttraumatic stress disorder and physical illness: results from clinical and epidemiologic studies. Ann NY Acad Sci 2004;1032: 141-153.

[121] David D, Woodward C, Esquenazi J, Mellman TA. Comparison of comorbid physical illnesses among veterans with PTSD and veterans with alcohol dependence. Psychiatr Serv 2004;55: 82-85.

[122] Shemesh E, Yehuda R, Milo O, Dinur I, Rudnick A, Vered Z, Cotter G. Posttraumatic stress, nonadherence and adverse outcome in survivors of a myocardial infarction. Psychosom Med 2004;66: 521-526.

[123] Baker DG, Ekhator NN, Kasckow JW, Dashevsky B, Horn PS, Bednarik L, Gander ML, Von Känel R. Myocardial infarction and post-traumatic stress disorder: frequency, outcome, and atherosclerotic mechanisms. Eur J Cardiovasc Prev 2006;13: 165-172.

[124] Reichlin S. Neuroendocrine-immune interactions. N Engl J Med 1993;329: 1246-1253.

[125] Spangelo BL, Judd A, Call G, Zumwalt J, Gorospe WC. Role of the cytokines in the hypothalamic-pituitary-adrenal and gonadal axes. Neuroimmunomodulation 1995;2: 299-312.

[126] Haddad JJ, Saadé NE, Safieh-Garabedian B. Cytokines and neuro-immune-endocrine interactions: a role for the hypothalamic-pituitary-adrenal revolving axis. J Neuroimmunol 2002; 133(1-2): 1-19

[127] Ransohoff RM, Benveniste EN. Cytokines and the CNS(second ed.) UK: CRC Press LLC; 2005.

[128] Faith RE, Murgo AJ, Good RA, Plotnikoff NP. Cytokines: stress and immunity (second ed.) UK: CRC Press LLC; 2006.

[129] Pace TW, Heim CM. A short review on the psychoneuroimmunology of posttraumatic stress disorder: from risk factors to medical comorbidities.Brain Behav Immun 2011;25(1): 6-13.

[130] O'Brien SM, Scully P, Scott LV, Dinan TG. Cytokine profiles in bipolar affective disorder: focus on acutely ill patients. J Affect Disord 2006;90(2-3): 263-267.

[131] Fan X, Goff DC, Henderson DC. Inflammation and schizophrenia. Expert Rev Neurother 2007;7(7): 789-796.

[132] Gardner A, Boles RG. Beyond the serotonin hypothesis: mitochondria, inflammation and neurodegeneration in major depression and affective spectrum disorders. Prog Neuropsychopharmacol Biol Psychiatry 2011;35(3): 730-743.

[133] Sim RB, Laich A. Serine proteases of the complement system. Biochem Soc Trans 2000;28: 545-550.

[134] Cole DS, Morgan BP. Beyond lysis: how complement influences cell fate. Clin Sci 2003; 104(5): 455-466.

[135] Nauta AJ, Roos A, Daha MR. A regulatory role for complement in innate immunity and autoimmunity. Int Arch Allergy Immunol 2004;134(4): 310-323.

[136] Sakamoto M, Fujisawa Y, Nishioka K. Physiologic role of the complement system in host defense, disease, and malnutrition. Nutrition 1998;14(4): 391-398.

[137] Volankis JE, Frank MM: The human complement system in health and disease. New York: Mircel Dekker Inc; 1998.

[138] Mollnes TE, Song W-C, Lambris JD: Complement in inflammatory tissue damage and disease. Trends Immunol Today 2002;23(2): 61-66.

[139] Morgan BP, Gasque P, Singhrao SK, Piddlesden SJ. The role of complement in disorders of the nervous system. Immunopharmacology 1997;38(1-2): 43-50.

[140] Yasojima K, Schwab C, McGeer EG, McGeer PL. Up-regulated production and activation of the complement system in Alzheimer's disease brain. Amer J Pathol 1999;154(3): 927-936.

[141] Gasque P, Neal JW, Singhrao SK, McGreal EP, Dean YD,Van BJ, Morgan BP. Roles of the complement system in human neurodegenerative disorders: pro-inflammatory and tissue remodeling activities. Mol Neurobiol 2002;25(1): 1-17.

[142] Francis K, Van Beek J, Canova C, Neal JW, Gasque P. Innate immunity and brain inflammation: the key role of complement. Expert Rev Mol Med 2003;5(15): 1-19.

[143] Van Beek J, Elward K, Gasque P. Activation of complement in the central nervous system: roles in neurodegeneration and neuroprotection. Ann N Y Acad Sci 2003;992: 56-71.

[144] Boyajyan A, Zakharyan R, Khoyetsyan A. Molecular and genetic indicators of aberrant immunity and apoptosis in schizophrenia. In: SumiyoshiT. (ed.) Schizophrenia Research: Recent Advances. USA: Nova Science Publishers Inc; 2012, p183-240.

[145] Maes M, Hendriks D, Van Gastel A, Demedts P, Wauters A, Neels H, Janca A, Scharpé S: Effects of psychological stress on serum immunoglobulin, complement, and acute phase protein concentrations in normal volunteers. Psychoneuroendocrinology 1997;22: 397-409.

[146] Burns V, Edwards K, Ring C, Drayson M, Carroll D. Complement cascade activation after an acute psychological stress task. Psychosomatic Medicine 2008;70: 387-396.

[147] Doods AW, Sim RB. Complement. A practical approach. Practical Approach series, Oxford: Oxford University Press Inc; 1997.

[148] Morgan P. Complement methods and protocols. Methods of Molecular Biology series. Totowa, New Jersey: Humana Press Inc; 2000.

[149] Hovhannisyan LP, Mkrtchyan GM, Boyajyan AS, Sukiasian SH. Immune complexes and complement classical cascade in posttraumatic stress disorder. Russ Biomed J 2008;9(2): 269-274. http://www.medline.ru/public/art/tom9/art023pdf.phtml

[150] Hovhannisyan L, Mkrtchyan G, Boyajyan A, Sukiasian S, Kalashyan A. Classical and alternative pathways complement activity and circulating immune complexes in patients with post-traumatic stress disorder. Scandinavian Journal of Immunology 2008;68(2): 204-205.

[151] Hovhannisyan LP, Mkrtchyan GM, Sukiasian SH, Ambardzumyan MK, Avetisyan GV, Boyajyan AS. Complement as a pathogenic factor in posttraumatic stress. Biol J Armenia 2009;61(1): 48-53.

[152] Hovhannisyan LP, Mkrtchyan GM, Sukiasyan SH, Boyajyan AS. Alterations in the complement cascade in post-traumatic stress disorder. Allergy, Asthma and Clinical Immunology 2010;6:3doi:10.1186/1710-1492-6-3.

[153] Gander ML, von Kanel R. Myocardial infarction and post-traumatic stress disorder: frequency, outcome, and atherosclerotic mechanisms. Eur J Cardiovasc Prev Rehabil 2006;13: 165-172.

[154] Schifferli JA, Ng YC, Peters DK. The role of complement and its receptor in the elimination of immune complexes. N Eng J Med 1986;315: 488-495.

[155] Moulds JM. Introduction to antibodies and complement. Transfus Apher Sci 2009;40(3): 185-188.

[156] Ng YC, Schifferli JA, Walport MJ. Immune complexes and erythrocyte CR1 (complement receptor type 1): effect of CR1 numbers on binding and release reactions. Clin Exp Immunol 1988;71: 481-485.

[157] Hebert LA. The clearance of immune complexes from the circulation of man and other primates. Am J Kidney Dis 1991;17:352-361.

[158] Thornton BP, Větvicka V, Ross GD. Natural antibody and complement-mediated antigen processing and presentation by B lymphocytes. J Immunol 1994;152(4): 1727-1737.

[159] Theofilopoulos AN. Evaluation and clinical significance of circulating immune complexes. Prog Clin Immunol 1980;4: 63-106.

[160] McDougal JS, McDuffie FC. Immune complexes in man: detection and clinical significance. Adv Clin Chem 1985;24: 1-60.

[161] Konstantinova N.A. Immune complexes and tissue damage. Moscow: Medicine; 1996.

[162] Shmagel KV, Chereshnev VA. Molecular bases of immune complex pathology. Biochemistry (Mosc) 2009;74(5): 469-479.

[163] Burut DF, Karim Y, Ferns GA. The role of immune complexes in atherogenesis. Angiology 2010;61(7): 679-689.

[164] Theofilopoulos AN, Dixon FJ. Immune complexes in human diseases. Am J Pathol 1980, 100(2): 529–594.

[165] Hovsepyan M, Boyajyan A, Aivazyan V, Mayilyan K, Guevorkyan A, Mamikonyan A. Concentration of circulating immune complexes and dopamine-hydroxylase activity in the blood of patients with diabetes mellitus type 1 at the late stages of the disease progression. Diabetes Mellitus (Mosc.) 2002;17(4): 44-45.

[166] Ovsepyan MR, Boyadjyan AS, Mamikonyan AA, Gevorkyan AA. Circulating immune complexes at the late stages of diabetes mellitus. Immunology (Mosc) 2004;25: 375

[167] Tarnacka B, Gromadzka G, Czlonkowska A. Increased circulating immune complexes in acute stroke: the triggering role of Chlamydia pneumoniae and cytomegalovirus. Stroke 2002;33(4): 936-940.

[168] Arakelian A, Boiadzhian A, Pogosian A, Bakunts G, Sil'vanian G, Egiian L. Circulating immune complexes in ischemic and hemorrhagic strokes. Zh Nevrol Psikhiatr Im S. S. Korsakova 2003;8: 44-47.

[169] Boiadzhian AS, Arakelova EA, Arakelian AA, Avetisian GV, Aivazian VA, Manucharian GG, Mkrtchian GM, Sim RB, Willis AK. Circulating immune complexes in families with positive history of ischemic stroke. Zh Nevrol Psikhiatr Im S. S. Korsakova 2007;21: 43-46.

[170] Hovhannisyan LP. Circulating immune complexes as possible inflammatory markers in posttraumatic stress disorder. Med Sci Armenia 2010;50(4): 69-75.

[171] Grunnet LG, Aikin R, Tonnesen MF, Paraskevas S, Blaabjerg L, Størling J, Rosenberg L, Billestrup N, Maysinger D, Mandrup-Poulsen T. Proinflammatory cytokines activate the intrinsic apoptotic pathway in beta-cells. Diabetes 2009;58(8): 1807-1815.

[172] Haanen C, Vermes I. Apoptosis and inflammation. Mediators of Inflammation 1995;4(1): 5-15.

[173] Savill J. Apoptosis in resolution of inflammation. J Leukocyte Biol 1997;61: 375-380.

[174] Chae JJ, Komarow HD, Cheng J, Wood G, Raben N, Liu PP, Kastner DL. Targeted disruption of pyrin, the FMF protein, causes heightened sensitivity to endotoxin and a defect in macrophage apoptosis. Mol Cell 2003;11(3) :591-604.

[175] Fantuzzi G. Adipose tissue, adipokines, and inflammation. J Allergy Clin Immunol 2005;115(5): 911-919.

[176] Parsey MV, Kaneko D, Shenkar R, Abraham E. Neutrophil apoptosis in the lung after hemorrhage or endotoxemia: apoptosis and migration are independent of interleukin-1β. Chest 1999;116: 67S-68S

[177] Jimenez MF, Watson RW, Parodo J, Evans D, Foster D, Steinberg M, Rotstein OD, Marshall JC. Dysregulated expression of neutrophil apoptosis in the systemic inflammatory response syndrome. Arch Surg 1997;132: 1263-1269.

[178] Li Z, Sheng M. Caspases in synaptic plasticity. Mol. Brain 2012;14(5): 15.

[179] Chan SL, Mattson MP. Caspase and calpain substrates: roles in synaptic plasticity and cell death. J Neurosci Res 1999;58: 167–190.

[180] Gilman CP, Mattson MP. Do apoptotic mechanisms regulate synaptic plasticity and growth-cone motility? Neuromolecular Med 2002;2(2): 197-214.

[181] Mahan AL, Ressler KJ. Fear conditioning, synapticplasticity and the amygdala: implications for posttraumatic stress disorder. Trends Neurosci 2012;35(1): 24-36.

[182] Duman RS. Pathophysiology of depression: the concept of synaptic plasticity. Eur Psychiatry 2002;17(3): 306-310.

[183] Hart J, Kimbrell T, Fauver P, Cherry BJ, Pitcock J, Booe LQ, Tillman G, Freeman TW. Cognitive dysfunctions associated with PTSD: evidence from World War II prisoners of war. J Neuropsychiatry Clin Neurosci 2008;20: 309-316.

[184] Moore SA. Cognitive abnormalities in posttraumatic stress disorder. Curr Opin Psychiatry 2009; 22(1): 19-24.

[185] Boersma HH, Kietselaer BL, Stolk LM, Bennaghmouch A, Hofstra L, Narula J, Heidendal GA, Reutelingsperger CP. Past, present, and future of Annexin A5: from protein discovery to clinical applications. JNM 2005;46(12): 2035-2050.

[186] Brose N. Altered complexin expression in psychiatric and neurological disorders: cause or consequence? Mol Cells 2008;25(1): 7-19.

Chapter 6

Understanding the Causes of Reduced Startle Reactivity in Stress-Related Mental Disorders

Kevin D. Beck and Jennifer E. Catuzzi

Additional information is available at the end of the chapter

1. Introduction

Many questions have plagued the study of the etiology and subsequent treatment of mental illness. In part, it is simply because, as far as we know, some mental illnesses are somewhat unique to the human condition. Moreover, clinical studies have produced many different results concerning potential biomarkers for conditions such as post-traumatic stress disorder (PTSD) and major depressive disorder (MDD). In this chapter, we review how we approached modeling a specific behavioral condition, suppression of the startle reflex, by examining whether one of two commonly associated peripheral biomarkers of anxiety and depression could potentially cause this rather specific symptom. The two peripheral systems under investigation were the hypothalamic-pituitary-adrenal (HPA) axis and the peripheral pro-inflammatory immune response, both of which have been implicated as a vulnerability factor, causal factor, or resultant (perpetuating) effect of PTSD and MDD.

Our general theory is that peripheral endocrine and immune signals, measured to be abnormal in patients with either PTSD or MDD (as well as other mental disorders), are actually perpetuating the behavioral features of these disorders. At the same time, if an individual has an immunosensitivity or has an overactive adrenal gland, s/he would be more likely to experience some of the symptoms associated with one of the particular mental illnesses. This may then lead the brain to compensate for those peripheral abnormalities, but, at the same time, cause other imbalances, which lead to the experience of a decline into mental illness. Thus, treating these peripheral markers as part of the "mental" disorder may be quite beneficial in normalizing certain aspects of the diagnosed abnormal behavior.

2. The startle reflex and mental health

2.1. The startle reflex as an assessment tool

One of the major impediments to the mechanistic study of mental illness is establishing analogs of the abnormal behaviors expressed in humans in animal models, especially in sub-primate species. This has led some to adopt reflex-based measures such that the face and construct validity of the behavior change can be readily translated between the model and patient populations. Consequently, a popular measures for the study of anxiety disorders has been the potentiation of the startle reflex; however, there is growing evidence that a dampening of the startle response may be indicative of changes in physiology that underlie different mental disorders.

The startle reflex comprises a 3-synaptic sensory-motor neuronal pathway that serves as a defensive behavioral response to abrupt, usually intense, stimuli. The acoustic startle response (ASR) is the most commonly used form for studying this reflex. As shown in Figure 1, the primary ASR circuit begins with neurons in the cochlear nerve, transmitting the representation of the acoustic stimulus from the cochlea of the inner ear to the cochlear nucleus (in the brainstem). Efferent pathways from the cochlear nucleus project to the nucleus reticularis pontis caudalis (PnC), in the pons, forming the second synapse in this reflex arc. The third synapse forms from the efferent projections from the PnC to various motor nuclei, through the recticulospinal spinal tracts to the muscles of the torso [1] and the muscles enervated by the facial nerve. These muscle enervations create a rapid cascade of near-immediate behavioral responses to abrupt acoustic stimuli, ranging from less than 10 ms to approximately 50 ms.

The ASR is modulated by several afferent connections originating from higher brain areas (midbrain, limbic, and cortical nuclei). At the level of the PnC, there are several inputs that can either enhance or inhibit the magnitude of an elicited ASR. In the area of fear and anxiety, the central amygdala and bed nucleus of the stria terminalis (BNST) are considered the 2 major excitatory modulation structures on this reflex [2]. Some have proposed that the BNST is the origin of anxiety-like behaviors whereas the nuclei of the amygdala are the origin of acute fear responses and explicit fear-learning [3, 4]. The amygdala is predominately associated with causing classically conditioned fear-potentiated ASRs [5], and, in fact, has been specifically shown not to have a role in startle inhibition, at least via a learned conditioned inhibitor [6]. On the other hand, the process known as pre-pulse inhibition of the startle reflex (PPI) has elucidated neural pathways that can inhibit the expression of the ASR. For instance, the substantial nigra pars retriculata (SNR), pedunculopontine tegmentum (PPT) and laterodorsal tegmental nuclei (LDT) have inhibitory influence upon the PnC, thus reducing the measured ASR [7-10]. These three mid-brain nuclei (inhibitory) receive projections from various forebrain areas, including the amygdala, BNST, and medial prefrontal cortex (mPFC). Thus, limbic system modulation of the ASR can occur through direct enervation of the PnC (excitatory) or indirect enervation through mid-brain nuclei.

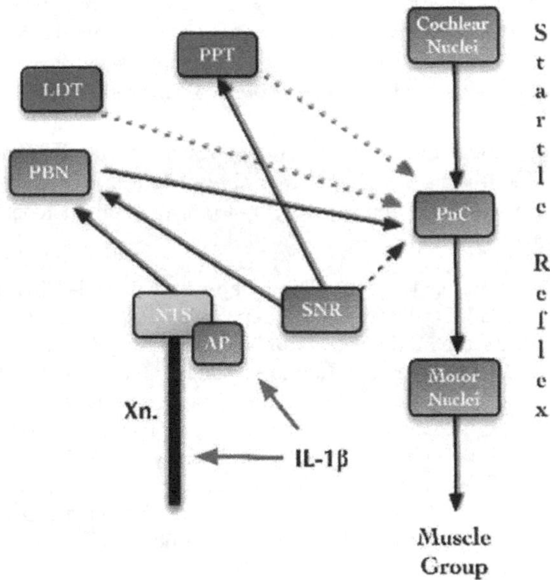

Figure 1. There are several nuclei within the midbrain/brainstem area that can directly modulate the intrinsic ASR circuit at the level of the nucleus reticularis pontis caudalis (PnC). Dashed red lines represent cholinergic inhibitory influences from the laterodorsal tegmental nuclei (LDT) and pedunculopontine tegmentum (PPT). Dashed black lines represent inhibitory GABAergic projections from the substantial nigra pars reticulata (SNR). A solid line from the parabrachial nucleus (PBN) is an example of a direct excitatory input to the PnC.

2.2. Abnormalities in the expression of the startle reflex in mental disorders

Over all other mental disorders, PTSD is associated with changes in the startle reflex. Commonly associated with exaggerated startle responses [11-14], higher or exaggerated startle reflex responses are a criteria symptom for the diagnosis of PTSD [15]. However, recent evidence suggests that this may not always be the case. In fact, others have reviewed the literature and found there are a significant number of reports where the startle responses in PTSD patients are not exaggerated [16]. More extreme, there are reports, albeit limited, where patients diagnosed with PTSD appeared to have blunted motor reflex responses to an acoustic stimulus [17, 18]. These populations had distinctive qualities that were different than those studies that had found enhanced startle reactivity in their PTSD patients. First, the one study was exclusively female [18] and the other had a majority of female subjects [17], suggesting there may be a sex difference in the presentation of ASR in females as a result of experiencing trauma. However, others have reported enhanced startle responses in a different population of women diagnosed with PTSD following automobile accidents [19]. Thus, a second distinction between the two studies that observed suppressed startle reactions, which should be considered, is that the trauma was specifically associated with being the target of violence [17, 18]. Although women with a PTSD diagnosis stemming from a prior rape have not always exhibited blunted startle responses [20], this discrepancy may be due to individual differences and/or methodological differences in being sensitive to such changes, as some have reported laterality effects in PTSD patients, notably of those having been raped in the past [21]. A third quality of at least one of these two reports is that the subjects also exhibited symptoms associated with major depressive disorder [18]. This suggests stressful experiences may not cause a uniform change in sensory reactivity, and the expression of the coping response to the trauma may have psychophysiological ramifications that are quite different, both in terms of effects upon sensory-motor responding to acoustic stimuli as well as the full expression of symptoms.

There is evidence that symptoms associated with depression may also include a blunted reaction to acoustic stimuli. Patients designated as "depressed", having either a diagnosis of MDD or a significantly higher score on the Beck Depression Inventory (with or without additional neurological conditions), have been reported to exhibit blunted reactivity to acoustic stimuli, either with or without manipulations of affect [22-26]. Similarly, there is also evidence that bipolar disorder (BPD), the occurrence of at least one manic or mixed manic episode over the course of a patient's lifetime, is characterized by blunted startle reactions as well, even during periods of remission [27]. A study by Carroll and colleagues found patients suffering from BPD exhibit attenuated baseline startle, most notably in those having experienced mixed episodes, not pure mania [28]. These data suggest there is a neurobiology of startle suppression that may provide critical insight to the underlying biological conditions that cause areas of the brain to improperly process information, in this case sensory-motor responses.

2.3. Animal models utilizing stress to dampen startle reactivity

Across the studies that have documented reductions in the expression of the startle reflex in rodents, the common-most feature is that the magnitude of the response is dampened following exposure to a stressor manipulation. Reduced startle amplitudes have been documented in rats following: repeated 20 min restraint [29]; inescapable tailshock [30-32]; predator exposure coupled with an intraperitoneal injection [33]; immune-challenge [34, 35], and a single session of footshocks [36]. Interestingly, despite some differences in methodology, inescapable tailshock [30], inescapable footshock [36], and predator exposure with injection [33], all showed reduction in ASR measurements that could *not* be attributable to enhanced habituation to the acoustic stimuli. Yet, studies utilizing inescapable tailshock (in females) *have* established that exposure to the stressor condition causes a change in startle responsivity (the magnitude of the measured startle responses), not startle sensitivity (the threshold to elicit a certain percentage of startle responses). Thresholds for eliciting ASRs are not increased in the shocked females; instead, the magnitudes of the elicited startle responses are lower [31, 32]. This suggests, at least for the female stress model, that the presumed increased inhibition upon the activity in the intrinsic ASR circuit is occurring through the motor response aspect of the reflex arc. The muscles are simply not as mobilized when this condition is induced. This model condition has been termed by some *stress-induced startle suppression* [32, 34].

There are significant differences in the temporal characteristics of these different startle-suppression models in rodents. Inescapable tailshock causes a reduction in startle magnitude in female rats that is evident hours within exposure [31, 32], possibly lasting up to a day later, when the bouts of shock are expanded to a few consecutive days [30]. The footshock-induced suppression of startle reactivity is evident 4 h following stressor exposure [36]. The immune-challenge models parallel these stressor manipulations by causing reductions in startle reactivity within a couple hours of administration of the challenge [34, 35]. Thus, one interpretation of these data is that painful stressors are causing changes in the peripheral immune system, which, in turn, dampen startle reactivity during the time of their activity [34], on the range of hours. Following this logic, when females were tracked 4 and 8 days following tailshock, reductions in startle reactivity in the stressor-exposed rats did not reach statistical significance [30]. In contrast, the predator-exposure + injection model shows immediate suppression following the stressor exposure, which continues to be present 1 week later [33]. In addition, it is evident both under dark and light conditions [33], suggesting the change in the startle response is not occurring due to a change in reactivity to other stimuli that are known to modulate startle reactivity, such as light-enhanced startle [37]. Thus, this observance suggests that changes in ASR magnitude may be extended beyond the acute effects of stressor exposure that could be attributed to the short-term effects of immune signaling that would be in response to the injection (or possibly even shock).

3. Peripheral mechanisms of reduced startle reactivity

3.1. Hypothalamic-Pituitary Adrenal (HPA)–axis

Two interrelated mechanisms have been proposed as potential causes of startle suppression, the first being glucocorticoid hormone reception. Adamec and colleagues showed the reduction of startle magnitudes following combined cat exposure and saline injection could be blocked by substituting the saline injection with the glucocorticoid receptor antagonists RU-486 [33]. We subsequently tried to induce the effect in our female rats by administering the synthetic glucocorticoid agonist, dexamethasone. Startle responses were assessed 2 and 4 h following dexamethasone administration. As shown in Figure 2, the dexamethasone did not appreciably change the magnitude of the elicited ASRs, nor did it affect the number of ASRs elicited (data not shown). These findings suggest that the reception of corticosterone at the glucorticoid receptor is not sufficient to reduce ASR magnitudes. One possibility is that RU-486 blocked the suppressed startle, in that model system, via a non-glucocorticoid mechanism, for example via progesterone receptor antagonism. A connection to progesterone will be discussed further below as it pertains to a pro-inflammatory response mechanism, in contrast to an anti-inflammatory glucocorticoid response, but this finding is supported by previous work that shows elevations in circulating corticosterone are not necessary for corticotrophin releasing hormone to increase ASR magnitudes, despite stimulating increased activity in the HPA-axis [38]. Likewise, the suppression of ASR magnitudes in Occidental low saccharine consuming rats is not recapitulated by substituting corticosterone administration for the shock exposure [36]. Therefore, a role of glucocorticoids in the suppression of ASR magnitudes may be limited.

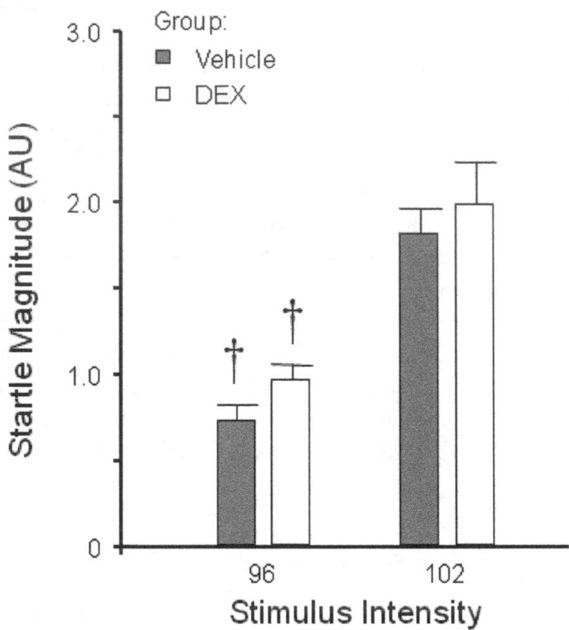

Figure 2. In order to increase binding at the glucocorticoid receptors, the synthetic glucocorticoid analog, dexamethasone, was administered s.c. (0.1 mg/kg) to female Sprague Dawley rats (n= 8-9). The magnitudes of the elicited ASRs only differed across the Stimulus Intensity, $F(1, 15) = 135.3$, $p < .001$, not drug administration. Data are collapsed over the 2 startle test sessions. A cross (†) represents within-group difference from the highest stimulus intensity ($p < .05$, Fishers LSD).

3.2. Pro-inflammatory cytokines

The second mechanism, which is intertwined with the HPA-axis, is the peripheral pro-inflammatory immune response. We first showed that a ovarian hormone-dependent suppression of startle magnitudes could be induced by a single injection of the pro-inflammatory cytokine interleukin (IL)-1β [34], an effect that appears to parallel that observed following tailshock [31]. This effect was later replicated in male rats using lipopolysaccharide (LPS) [35]. Still, peripherally released IL-1β elicits the release of glucocorticoids from the adrenal through stimulation of the vagus nerve, paraventricular nucleus of the hypothalamus, and pituitary gland, which provides an anti-inflammatory response to the pro-inflammatory signal [39-44]. In order to further delineate that pro-inflammatory cytokines, and not anti-inflammatory glucocorticoids, are necessary for stress-induced startle suppression, we compared the effect of inescapable tailshock upon the induction of ASRs in two strains of rats, specifically chosen because of their pro-inflammatory and glucocorticoid responsiveness to stressors. Low-glucocorticoid/high-pro-inflammatory releasing Lewis (LEW) rats [45-49] and high-glucocorticoid releasing Wistar-Kyoto (WKY) rats [50-52] were compared.

Females of each of these strains were exposed to inescapable tailshock and subsequently tested for startle reactivity 1 and 3 h later. If pro-inflammatory signaling, not anti-inflammatory glucocorticoid release is critical for eliciting startle suppression, then LEW rats would exhibit suppression of the ASR, and the WKY rats would not. As shown in Figure 3, this is the case. This suggest the suppression of startle responsivity in female rats is more likely due to an overactive pro-inflammatory cytokine signaling response, instead of an overactive anti-inflammatory glucocorticoid response via the HPA-axis.

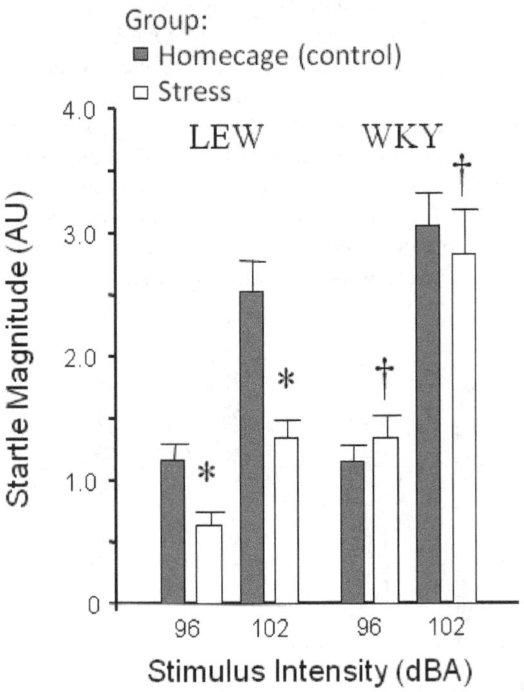

Figure 3. LEW rats exposed to the stressor differed from both their same-strain controls and the WKY groups on the measure of startle magnitude (responsivity). These impressions were confirmed by both main effects of Stimulus Intensity, $F(1, 36) = 285.0$, $p < .0001$, Strain, $F(1, 36) = 6.4$, $p < .02$, and Stressor exposure, $F(1, 36) = 5.3$, $p < .03$, as well as a marginal Strain x Stressor interaction, $F(1, 36) = 3.3$, $p < .07$. In addition to the expected differences in ASR magnitude due to Stimulus Intensity, $F(2, 72) = 186.5$, $p < .0001$, there were differences in the number of elicited startles across the two strains at the lowest stimulus intensity, with WKY rats having responded with more startles (4.5) than did the LEW rats (3.8) to 92 dBA stimulus. This impression was confirmed by a significant Strain x Stimulus Intensity interaction, $F(2, 72) = 3.0$, $p < .05$ (data not shown).

The hypothesis that pro-inflammatory cytokines are a necessary component in the suppression of startle responses following stress was further evaluated in the immune-sensitive Lewis rat strain by determining if elevations of peripheral IL-1β is sufficient to suppress startle reactivity in female rats. Startle responsivity has been found to be suppressed in female SD rats

[34], but, we questioned whether immune-sensitive Lewis rats would show either greater effect sizes in the suppression of the startle magnitudes and/or reduced startle sensitivity as well. As shown in Figure 4, both startle responsivity and sensitivity were reduced in female Lewis rats administered IL-1β. This confirms that pro-inflammatory signaling can influence both aspects of startle behavior, with sensitivity effects requiring a greater sensitivity to the pro-inflammatory signals or, possibly, greater elevations of the signal.

3.3. Prior immune challenge effects on stress-induced startle in SD rats

One consequence of the peripheral immune system having an effect on behavior, in this case sensory reactivity to acoustic stimuli, is that prior immune challenges may influence how future pro-inflammatory signaling or anti-inflammatory glucocorticoid responses influences behavior following stressor exposure. LPS is a commonly used endotoxin that elicits sickness behaviors due to a release of peripheral and central pro-inflammatory cytokines, followed by an increase in circulating glucocorticoids [53, 54]. Others have shown that immune challenges days prior to shock exposure causes a greater increase in glucocorticoid release in response to shocks [55, 56]; therefore, we used this known method of causing a sensitized glucocorticoid response to determine if a greater glucocorticoid release enhances or reduces the degree by which tailshock suppresses startle responsivity.

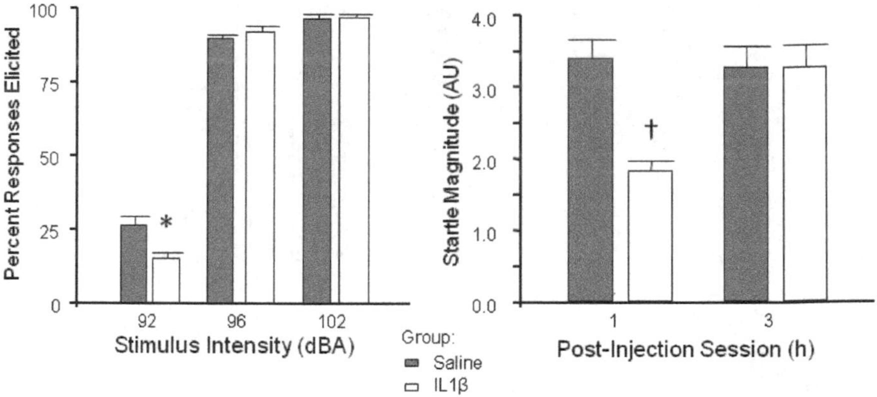

Figure 4. Female LEW rats (n = 16) exhibited significant differences in both startle sensitivity and startle responsivity measures following a single systemic injection of IL-1β (3 μg/kg, i.p.). Startle sensitivity was equally effected 1 and 3 h following administration and is shown collapsed over Session Time. Startle responsivity was only effected 1 h following administration; therefore, the 3 h time-point is not shown. An asterisk (*) represents a significant difference from saline-treated controls at the same stimulus intensity. A cross (†) represents a significant difference from saline-treated controls during the same test session (all $p < .05$, Fishers LSD).

We hypothesized that pro-inflammatory signaling causes stress-induced startle suppression; therefore, experiencing an immune challenge 3 days prior to shock would cause a sensitized anti-inflammatory release of glucocorticoids in response to inescapable shock, blocking the reduction of startle responsivity caused by the acute release of pro-inflammatory cytokines.

As expected, the number of startle responses elicited did not differ based on prior treatment but did differ across stimulus intensity (data not shown); however, prior exposure to LPS reduced the effectiveness of inescapable shock to attenuate startle magnitudes (see Figure 5). Although LPS has a short-term suppressing effect upon the startle response [35], it both causes an acute increase in pro-inflammatory cytokines (and sickness behaviors) followed by an increase in anti-inflammatory glucocorticoid signaling. This "priming" effect upon the anti-inflammatory glucocorticoid response to shock is a likely mechanism for "buffering" the behavior from being affected. Again, this suggests the glucocorticoid response may actually counteract the suppressive effects originating from peripheral pro-inflammatory cytokine signaling.

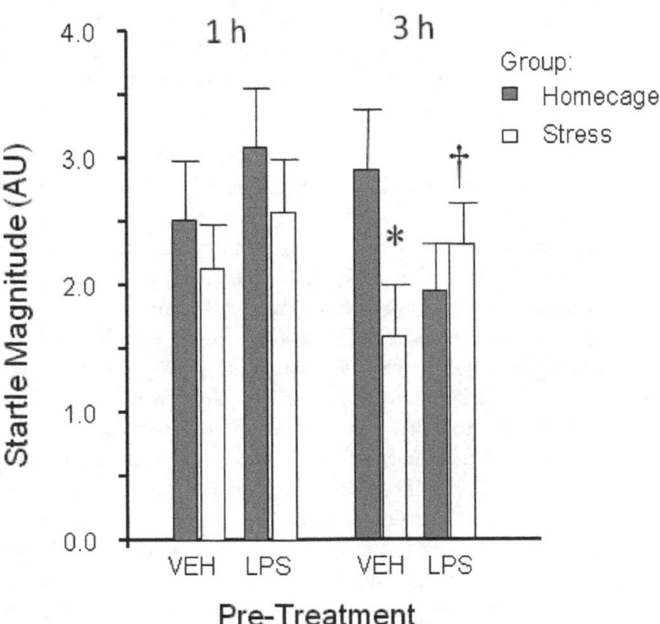

Figure 5. The expression of stress-induced startle suppression became evident 3 h following stressor exposure; however, this effect was blocked in those rats previously exposed to 30 μg/kg LPS (i.p.) 3 days earlier. These impressions were confirmed by a significant LPS x Stress x Session interaction, $F(1, 28) = 10.2$, $p < .005$. Hence, the pretreatment with LPS, which should have increased the glucocorticoid response to the inescapable tailshocks, blocked the suppression of startle responsivity following shock exposure. This suggests that prior experiences likely cause a more robust anti-inflammatory glucocorticoid response that actually *reduces* the influence of the peripheral immune pro-inflammatory immune response upon the areas of the brain capable of suppressing startle responsivity.

4. Central mechanisms of reduced startle reactivity

4.1. Neuroanatomy and endocrine modulation of startle suppression

As mentioned above, studies of pre-pulse inhibition of the ASR have elucidated neural circuitry that underlie the suppression of ASRs when they are immediately preceded by a salient auditory stimulus, for a review see [57]. Both the BNST and AMG have indirect projections to the PnC through the PPT [58]. Inputs from the PPT, LDT, and SNR to the PnC cause inhibition of the startle response [7, 9, 59, 60]. More specifically, it appears the magnocellular portion of the PnC has muscarinic receptors to receive the inhibitory cholinergic signal from PPT and LDT [61] and $GABA_B$ receptors receive the inhibitory signal from the SNR [62]. The question is whether these areas could provide more tonic inhibition of the ASR, outside of the attentional processes associated with PPI. For instance, it is known that lesions to the medial septum and the fimbra-fornix increase startle reactivity because these areas provide tonic inhibition upon the amygdala [63]; thus, removal of inhibition upon the amygdala increases tonic excitatory activity to the PnC (from the amygdala). In contrast, lesions to the noradrenergic cell bodies of the LC reduce startle response magnitudes, as these neurons probably serve a tonic excitation function upon the PnC [64]. Thus, there are circuits within the brain that are situated such that they could provide more tonic changes in the ASR.

Specific to the female startle-suppression model, a central mechanism that caused this change in reactivity should be influenced by the presence/absence of ovarian hormones [31, 32]. Ovarian hormones can have a significant impact on many of the neural structures associated with startle regulation. The cochlear nuclei [65], the nucleus accumbens [66], the hippocampus, [67] and the SNR [57] all exhibit changes in morphology, neurotransmission, and/or receptor expression with the presence of ovarian hormones. Yet, despite all these areas of influence, rodent studies usually do not find any differences in baseline startle reactivity across the estrus cycle or with hormone replacement [68, 69]; however, see [70] for an example of oral-contraceptive usage effecting baseline startle in women. When significant arousal or stress occurs in the rodents, however, the modulatory actions of ovarian hormones on startle become evident. For example, Toufexis and colleagues have shown the magnitude of CRH-enhanced startle is attenuated when progesterone levels are increased [71]. CRH is thought to enhance startle reactivity in the BNST via CRF1-type receptors [72-75]. The result is an increase in excitatory afferents signaling to the PnC [76]. One possibility is that progesterone, or its metabolite allopregnanolone, may decrease the excitatory signaling from the BNST to the PnC by increasing GABA inhibition in this structure [77]. However, in vitro, BNST CRF-1 receptors increase local GABA activity [78]. Thus, it appears that progesterone or allopregnanolone should facilitate the actions of CRH on startle, unless they act through different mechanisms within the BNST or outside of the BNST. On the other hand, progesterone also affects how IL-1β influences sexual receptivity [79], and both glucocorticoid receptor activation [77] and progesterone-induced changes in central neuroadrenergic activity [80] have been suggested to attenuate startle reactivity selectively in female rats. As shown in Figure 6, the administration of progesterone to ovariectomized rats appears to be necessary for IL-1β to suppress startle magnitudes. Thus, ovarian hormones are not sufficient to cause changes in startle reactivity in female rats. In fact, IL-1β appears to increase startle responsivity following estradiol pretreatment (17β-estradiol), whereas progesterone pretreatment sets the stage for IL-1β to suppress startle responsivity. Therefore, stress-induced startle suppression in female rats appears to necessitate a combination of the two factors, a peripheral pro-inflammatory immune response and the presence of progesterone.

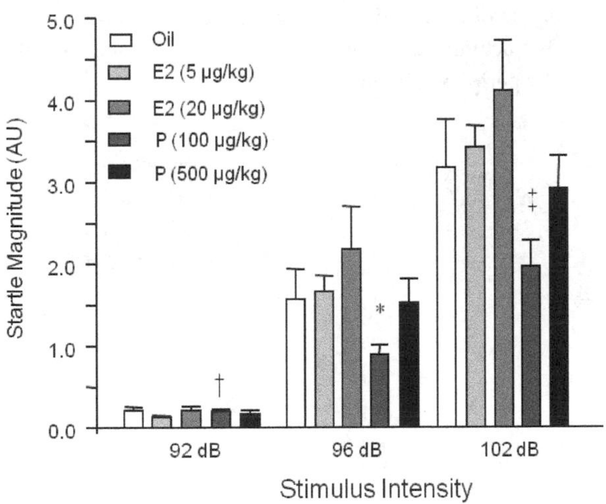

Figure 6. Startle sensitivity and responsiveness were assessed 2 h following IL-1β administration. Hormone treatment occurred 2 h prior to IL-1β injection. Differences in startles elicited (sensitivity) and the magnitudes of those elicited startle responses (responsivity) each were assessed via a 5 (Condition) x 3 (Stimulus Intensity) repeated measures ANOVA. No significant differences in startle sensitivity were detected (data not shown). However, a significant main effect of Stimulus Intensity, $F(2, 70) = 392.2$, $p < .001$ and a significant Condition x Stimulus Intensity interaction, $F[8, 70] = 2.1$, $p < .05$ were detected in the measure of startle responsivity (magnitude). An asterisk (*) represents a significant difference from all other groups. A single cross (†) represents a significant difference from the low estradiol dose group. A double cross (‡) represents a significant difference from both estradiol-treatment groups. All post-hoc tests used Fishers LSD ($p < .05$).

4.2. Evidence for limbic regulation of startle suppression

Peripheral IL-1β is known to have a significant impact on brain activity. Systemic IL-1 administration activates key afferent pathways in brainstem (lateral parabrachial nucleus and dorsomedial and ventrolateral medulla) and limbic system nuclei (BNST and central nucleus of the amygdala) [81]. In fact, peripheral IL-1β activates the amygdala and BNST more than i.c.v. administered IL-1β [82], probably because the vagal-mediated signals to these nuclei are more direct, to those nuclei via the NTS, than the diffusion of the IL-1β from the ventricles. Still, increasing peripheral IL-1β signaling increases NE and serotonin levels in these brain areas [83] and noradrenergic metabolism in the paraventricular nucleus of the hypothalamus (PVN), locus coeruleus (LC), and amygdala [83]. In fact, as the IL-1β dose is increased, the amount of NE metabolism increases linearly in the amygdala, lasting as much as an hour [83]. It should be noted, this was not tested in the BNST. Yet, stimulation of α-adrenergic receptors also attenuate startle responses and facilitate non-associative habituation of the startle response [84-88]. IL-1β affects activity in the LC in a dose dependent manner as well, with low doses inhibiting activity and higher doses causing excitation; a process mediated by CRH at the time of IL-1β release [89]. Further, when the exposure to painful stimuli is prolonged or LPS is used to cause a significant pro-inflammatory response, additional release of central IL-1β occurs, especially in the hypothalamus [90, 91]. These data suggest that activity in the limbic system, monoamine activity in particular, is significantly affected by peripheral immune signaling.

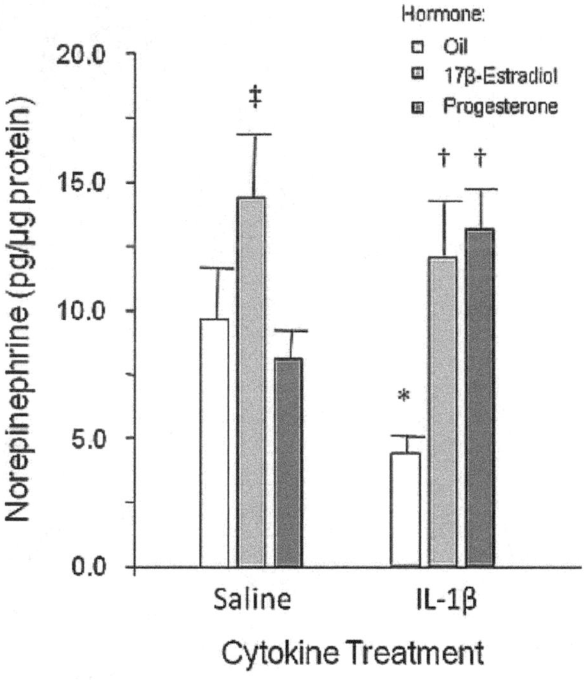

Figure 7. Significant effects of IL-1 treatment on NE levels in the BNST were observed in rats pretreated with progesterone (100 μg/kg, s.c.). This was confirmed by a significant Hormone x IL-1 interaction F (2, 42) = 4.5, p <.02. IL-1β treatment to oil-treated controls was associated with significantly lower NE levels than oil-treated saline-controls (*). IL-1β-administered rats, which were pretreated with either estradiol [20 μg/kg, s.c.) or progesterone, exhibited higher levels of NE compared to oil-pretreated rats that subsequently received IL-1β (†). In addition, the 2 hormone treated saline control conditions also differed from each other, with the estradiol-treated saline-controls exhibiting higher levels of NE than those pretreated with progesterone prior to saline administration (‡). All post-hoc tests utilized Fisher's LSD (p <.05).

Based on the above logic, we hypothesized that the reduction in ASR magnitude occurring as a result of IL-1β administration to progesterone-pretreated female rats could be associated with changes in the central noradrenergic activity in one of the known modulatory nuclei of the acoustic startle response. Therefore, we measured norepinephrine levels in brain tissue-punches from 4 brain areas: BNST, amygdala, medial prefrontal cortex (mPFC), and dorsal hippocampus. As stated above, both the BNST and cAMG have direct excitatory projections to the PnC and indirect inhibitory connections via the PPT. The medial prefrontal cortex projects to the primary startle circuit via the LDT, whereas the dorsal hippocampus was included as an area that is both reactive to stress and ovarian hormone manipulation, but it is actually several synapses removed from the PPT. As shown in Figure 7, differences due to hormone pretreatment and subsequent IL-1β administration were found in the BNST, not in any of the other 3 areas.

Green arrows from IL-1β¶

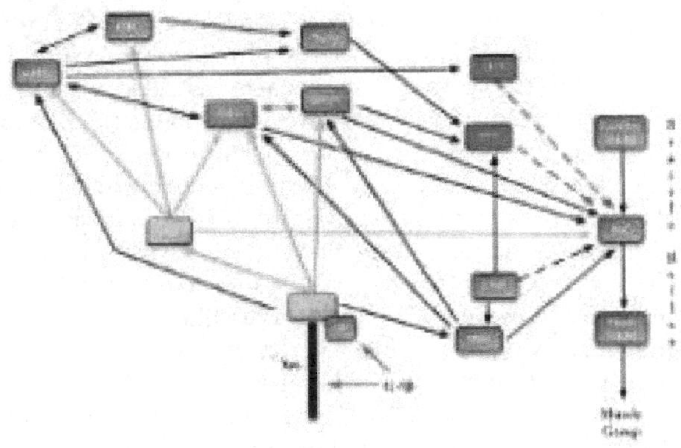

Figure 8. Beyond the direct connections of the brainstem/midbrain nuclei, there are many other nuclei that indirectly influence the modulation of the ASR. Graphically represented here are the noradrenergic projections (in blue) from the nucleus of the solitary tract (NTS) and locus coeruleus (LC) to the various nuclei of the limbic system that then modulate the ASR via the inhibitory brainstem/midbrain nuclei. Input to the NTS via either the from the vagus nerve (X n.) or diffusion of IL-1β across the blood-brain barrier in the nearby area postrema is necessary for the noradrenergic changes in the brain in response to peripheral pro-inflammatory cytokine signaling. As above, red lines denote cholinergic pathways, and dashed lines represent inhibitory circuits. The orange represents CRH-mediated neural circuits. See text for further details.

The role of the BNST in this cytokine-induced change in behavior is logical given recent work associating activity in this structure with changes in behavior associated with behavioral depression or sickness behavior. For example, an endotoxin-induced suppression of social interactions is both associated with increased activity in the BNST as well as reduced activity in the BNST when the suppressed behavior is blocked by IL-1ra [92]. Similarly, the behavioral depression exhibited in the forced-swim test can be reduced by stimulating the vagus nerve, leading to changes in brainstem nuclei activation (including the NTS) and also activation of the BNST [93]. Others have shown NE release is elevated with stressor exposure in the BNST, which is necessary for some stress-induced behaviors [94, 95]. With particular attention to the startle reflex, the BNST is commonly associated with enhancing startle reactivity [2, 96]. However, as shown in Figure 8), there is an inhibitory pathway from the BNST to the PnC via the PPT that has been examined as a cholinergic mechanism for eliciting PPI [97, 98]. Further, PPI has been shown to fluctuate over the estrus cycle, while not being sensitive to apomorphine disruption, implicating a non-dopaminergic mechanism for these hormone-induced changes in female pre-pulse inhibition, which could rule-out a role of the substantia nigra in this process [68]. In addition, the changes in measured NE levels in the BNST are consistent with previous studies citing peripheral IL-1β administration as a trigger for central noradrenergic activity [82, 99].

There is evidence that could suggest a connection between the known effects of peripheral cytokine activity upon brain noradrenergic activity (most reported males) and an ovarian hormone influence upon these processes. For one, there is growing information pertaining to ovarian hormone influences on noradrenergic activity initiated from the NTS. Many of the brainstem noradrenergic nuclei, including the NTS, exhibit cyclic changes in estrogen and progesterone receptors [100]. Removal of ovarian hormones with or without hormone replacement particularly has a significant impact on NTS physiology. Specifically, the mRNA for prolactin-releasing peptide (PrRP) in noradrenergic neurons is decreased by ovariectomy and increased with subsequent replacement of either estradiol or progesterone [101]. Although the PrRP mRNA levels are reported to not change significantly across the estrus cycle in the NTS, an inspection of the data suggests the levels are a bit higher during proestrus [102]. PrRP labeling in the NTS is also preferentially sensitive to painful stressors, such as tailshock [103]. Estradiol has also been reported to increase neural inhibition in the NTS [104]. These data suggest ovarian hormone influences on NE NTS physiology could occur through changes in the regulation of a co-expressing neuropeptide. This could serve a filtering function for the vagal activity representing immune activity changes in the periphery, as the NTS projects its NE efferent connections to key areas involved in arousal and sensory reactivity, such as the BNST, AMG, hypothalamus, and parabrachial nucleus [105]. For example, core body temperature increases from peripheral IL-1β occur for a longer period of time during proestrus (compared to diestrus) apparently do to the actions of progesterone [106]. Although it is clear hypothalamic cyclooxygenase is the necessary mechanism for this effect [107] the noradrenergic input to the hypothalamus is required and may be changed as well [108]. Therefore, there are anatomical and pharmacological reasons to link NTS noradrenergic projections to the BNST as the primary pathway by which changes in vagal activity could influence startle responsivity through known inhibitory circuitry.

Other possible mechanism for startle suppression could occur as a cascade of effects that begin with the hormone-specific effects upon NE in the brain, but end with non-specific hormonal influences upon 5-HT. NE was shown above to be changed in the BNST following systemic increases in IL-1β, confirming the results of others showing noradrenergic activity increases within 30 minutes of a peripheral injection of IL-1β and may last 2 hours [109, 110]. Importantly, as proposed above, the effect of systemic IL-1β injections on brain NE in rodents is dependent upon transmission in the vagus nerve [111]. The effects of peripheral IL-1β on 5-HT are quite different in terms of timing, route, and influence of ovarian hormones. First the increases observed in brain serotonin metabolism are evident 2-4 h following IL-1β administration and, at least in male rats, are reported to be less region specific (compared to NE activity changes) [110]. In addition, the effects of peripheral IL-1β on brain 5-HT are not dependent upon the vagus nerve in male mice but neither are the effects upon brain NE activity [112]. Thus, it is not known if 5-HT requires the same pathway as IL-1β to effect central 5-HT activity, but the difference in the temporal cascade would suggest such a difference is logical. Further, as shown in Figure 9, the same peripheral IL-1β injections that elicited a hormone-dependent change in BNST NE levels caused an increase in 5-HT activity in both estradiol and progesterone-treated female rats. This somewhat conforms to the data previously describing less specificity in the upregulation of 5-HT activity, although we did not observe this pattern beyond the BNST.

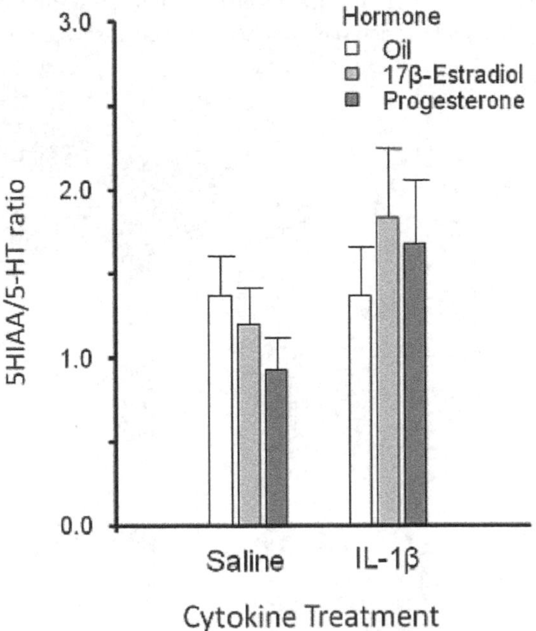

Figure 9. Serotonin activity (5HIAA/5HT ratio) appears to be increased in the BNST of hormone-pretreated OVX female rats 2 h after a systemic injection of IL-1β, as suggested by a marginal effect of IL-1β, $F(1, 42) = 3.6$, $p < .06$.

5. Immune mechanisms following the acute pro-inflammatory response: Recovery or maintenance?

5.1. Recovery of startle responsivity

The peripheral immune system also has counter-inflammation mechanisms that could also be potential mechanisms for what appears to be a pro-inflammatory cytokine-mediated effect. Thus, another response to pro-inflammatory cytokine release, is the increase in the endogenous IL-1 receptor antagonist (IL-1ra), which has been shown to attenuate the reductions in food-intake elicited by systemic administration of LPS or IL-1β [113]. Our hypothesis was that elevations in IL-1ra, from systemic administration, would counteract the effects of IL-1β. Thus, IL-1ra was administered systemically, followed by an assessment of startle reactivity 1 and 3 h later. As shown in Figure 10, the peripheral immune mechanism for stifling the pro-inflammatory response of IL-1β is sufficient to increase startle sensitivity. This suggests the nervous system is responsive to elevated acute pro-inflammatory signaling, suppressing startle, and elevations in the counter-active IL-1ra, increasing sensitivity to acoustic stimuli. These interactions illustrate the constant inter-relationship between the peripheral immune system and the nervous system regulation of sensory-motor activity.

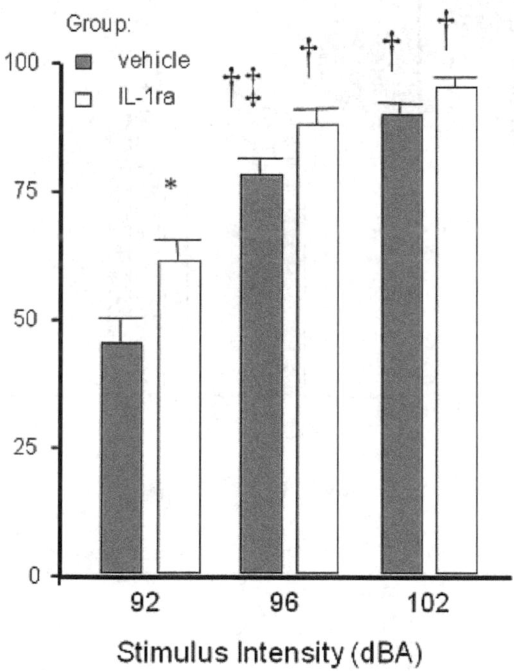

Figure 10. Startle magnitudes in female SD rats (n = 7) were not affected by the administration of IL-1ra (10μg/kg); however, ASRs were elicited more often following the administration of IL-1ra. These impressions were confirmed by a significant main effect of Drug $F(1, 12) = 9.7$, $p < .01$. The higher sensitivity to the stimuli was superimposed upon the general difference in elicited startles across the three intensities, as reflected by a main effect of Stimulus Intensity, $F(2, 24) = 67.4$, $p < .0001$. An asterisk (*) represents a significant between-group difference from the vehicle-treated controls at the same intensity. A cross (†) represents a significant within-subject difference from the lowest intensity, and a double cross (‡) represents a significant within-subject difference from the highest intensity (all $p < .05$, Fishers LSD).

5.2. Immune influences on serotonin synthesis: A possible central mechanism of continued suppression?

Serotonin (5-HT) is an essential modulator of the startle reflex and disruption of serotonin synthesis and metabolism has been shown to result in startle suppression. As shown in Figure 11, during the synthesis of serotonin, L-tryptophan is converted to 5-hydroxytryptophan (5-HTP) by the enzyme tryptophan hydroxylase. In a subsequent reaction, 5-HTP is converted to 5-HT by the enzyme L-aromatic amino acid decarboxylase. Disruption to any part of the 5-HT synthesis pathway is capable of reducing whole brain levels of serotonin resulting in unique abnormalities to the startle reflex. For example, when normal fasted women were tested after having ingested a tryptophan-free amino-acid mixture, the result was lower ASR magnitudes compared to those that received a mixture with L-tryptophan in its contents [114]. When a similar study was conducted in men, a non-significant trend for the same effect appears evident, although it was represented in the analysis as a failure to obtain significant PPI [115]. Alternatively, increasing tryptophan catabolism has also shown to affect PPI. Increasing levels of kynurenine, the first product of tryptophan degradation via indoleamine2, 3-dioxygenase, disrupts PPI in male Sprague-Dawley Rats [116]. Thus, the balance of serotonin and kynurenine is a likely secondary mechanism the body uses to modulate startle sensitivity and responsivity to stimuli.

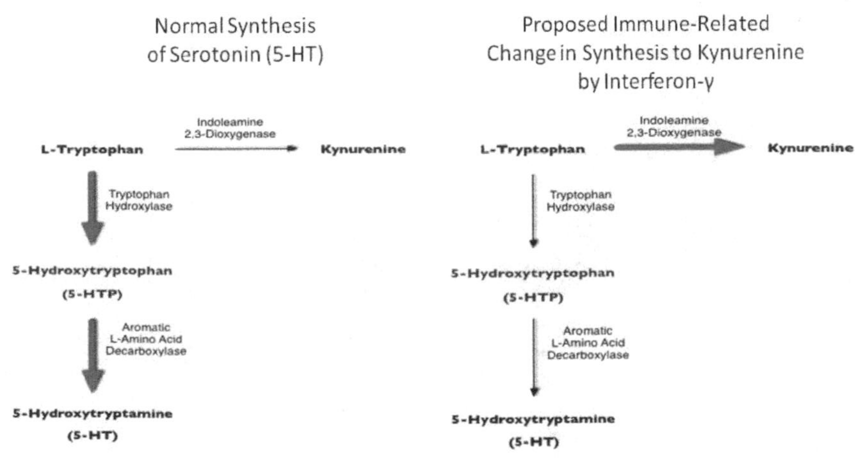

Figure 11. The normal synthesis of serotonin (5-HT) involves the metabolism of tryptophan to 5-hydroxytryophan by tryptophan hydroxylase; however, in the presence of interferon-γ, another, competing enzyme, indolamine1,3-dioxygenase is upregulated. The result of this shift in the metabolism of tryptophan towards the formation of kynurenine is a reduction in the amount available for metabolism towards the formation of serotonin (i.e. serotonin depletion).

In addition to exhibiting reduced startle responses [18] women exhibiting PTSD, linked to previous intimate partner violence, also exhibit greater circulating levels of interferon (INF)-

γ [117]. INF-γ is a downstream Th-1 mediated signal from the pro-inflammatory IL-1β signal and is a potent inhibitor of 5-HT synthesis, decreasing the amount of tryptophan available for 5-HT production. In the presence of IFN-γ, tryptophan is shunted to kynurenic acid synthesis by increasing activity of indoleamine2, 3-dioxygenase [118]. An intermediary signal between IL-1β and INF-γ is IL-2. Female rats treated with IL-1ra (to combat the induction of EAE) exhibit an attenuated IL-2 response [119], which would, presumably, decrease INF-γ signaling (see Figure 12). There is limited experimental evidence that has focused upon delineating INF-γ or IL-2 effects on startle reactivity in rats, and those that have been conducted use an early development administration paradigm to assess later changes on behavior (e.g. [120]). However, one study conducted in mice did access acute IL-2 effects upon startle reactivity and reported no change in behavior [121]. Unfortunately, that study did not test more than one time-point and only utilized male mice.

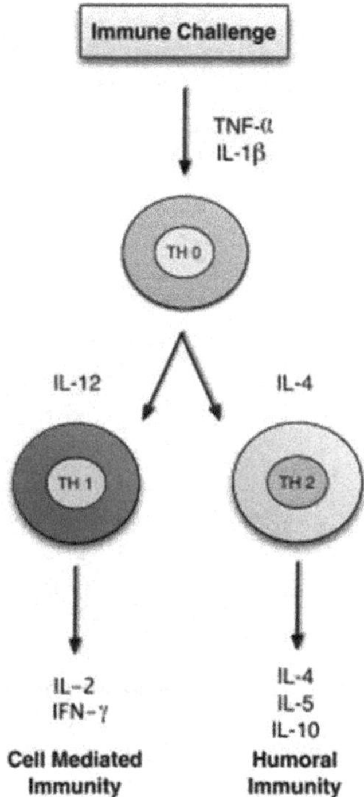

Figure 12. The initiation of an inflammatory response begins with the non-specific macrophage pro-inflammatory response (Th0), which then diverges into either a Th1 (cell-based) or Th2 (humoral-mediated) response. There is evidence that suggests ovarian hormones may influence the path of the subsequent immune cascade from the Th0 response. To date, the Th1 response has been more intently studied for its possible role in effecting behavior (i.e. causing changes in behavior).

Given the lack of data pertaining to IFN-γ effects upon startle sensitivity and responsivity, we conducted a study focusing on determining whether IFN-γ could change ASR sensitivity or responsivity. As stated above, LEW rats exhibit greater pro-inflammatory responses to infection than do other strains; therefore, we tested whether acute administration of IFN-γ is sufficient to reduce startle reactivity, presumably from reducing serotonin availability. Although still preliminary, our results suggest IFN-γ may have a bi-potential effect on startle sensitivity. The higher dose of IFN-γ caused an apparent decrease in the percentage of startles elicited 1.5 h following injection, whereas the lower dose caused significantly more startles to be elicited than the high dose (see Figure 13). This is an important distinction, for it suggests that reduced startle responding due to IFN-γ (and possibly low serotonin tone) is due to a decrease in the ability to sense a startling stimulus, rather than the ability to mount the physical response (although there are trends suggesting that responsivity may be decreased as well with higher doses). Hence, there may be more than a hypothetical link between stress, IL-1 release, and an identified difference in basal immune functioning in a population of women with PTSD that have also been described to have blunted startle responses. There may be instances where the downstream Th1-response is elevated, thus causing a seemingly similar "blunting" of the ASR but the suppression is different in form and occurs through different neural pathways.

6. Clinical applications

The suppression of startle reactions has only gained significant attention in the past decade, and, as researchers have looked for *changes* in startle responses (not just exaggerations), suppression has been observed in anxiety disorders (i.e. PTSD), MDD, and BPD. However, what does it mean when a specific, directional change in a reflex behavior is observed across these different diagnoses? The answer may lie in what is generally called *comorbidity*.

When one considers stress-related mental disorders, typically, anxiety disorders, MDD, BPD, and maybe even schizophrenia are cited as examples, but how distinct are anxiety disorders from MDD or MDD from BPD? In all cases, there is an overlap of various symptoms that could be experienced with any of these diagnoses. The DSM clinical criteria do provide some flexibility in categorizing subjects into the different classes of disorders. What that allows for are physiological conditions that are not specific to just one of these classes, and chronic or phasic abnormalities in the activities of the peripheral immune system could be common in some patients that meet the criteria for PTSD, the non-mania phase of BPD, or even MDD.

For example, there is a growing body of literature that suggests abnormal immune system signaling may be at the core of BPD. Several studies have shown abnormalities in the cytokine profiles of BPD patients, with differences present in both depressed and manic subpopulations [122-124]. Multiple studies have shown a characteristic increase in TNF-α among both bipolar depressed and manic patients [122, 123], whereas patients suffering from bipolar mania commonly exhibit decrease in IL-1β, IL-2, and IFN-γ. When stimulated with LPS, a common procedure used to model behavioral depression in animals, the monocytes from non-lithium treated patients exhibit a decrease in the production of IL-1β and an increase in IL-6, compared to healthy controls. This abnormality was shown to be reversed in lithium treatment patients [125]. This suggests a by-product of lithium administration may be an influence on the pro-inflammatory response signals in the periphery. Additionally, Boufidou and colleges found that lithium is capable of down regulating the production of IL-2, IL-6, IL-10 and IFN-γ from peripheral blood lymphocytes in BPD patients, and a similar down regulation of pro-inflammatory cytokines was observed in previously non-medicated BDP after three months of lithium treatment [126]. These data further implicate a peripheral immune mechanism for BPD that is normalized by lithium treatment.

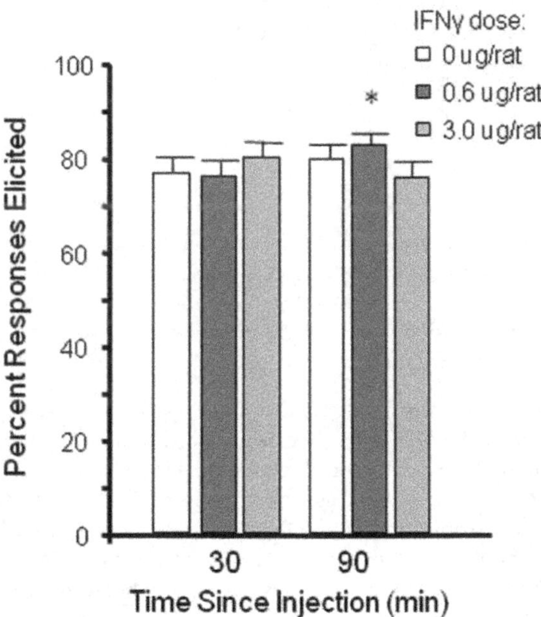

Figure 13. Startle sensitivity and responsivity were assessed 30 and 90 min following an acute systemic injection of IFN-γ (n = 16). Startle sensitivity was significantly altered by the specific dose administered. The low dose showed an increase in elicited startles over time, whereas the high dose showed a reduction in elicited startles over time, IFNγ x Session F (2, 29)= 3.3, p <.05. An asterisk represents a significant difference in the low-dose group at the 90 min test as compared to the same time high-dose and the 30-min low-dose test.

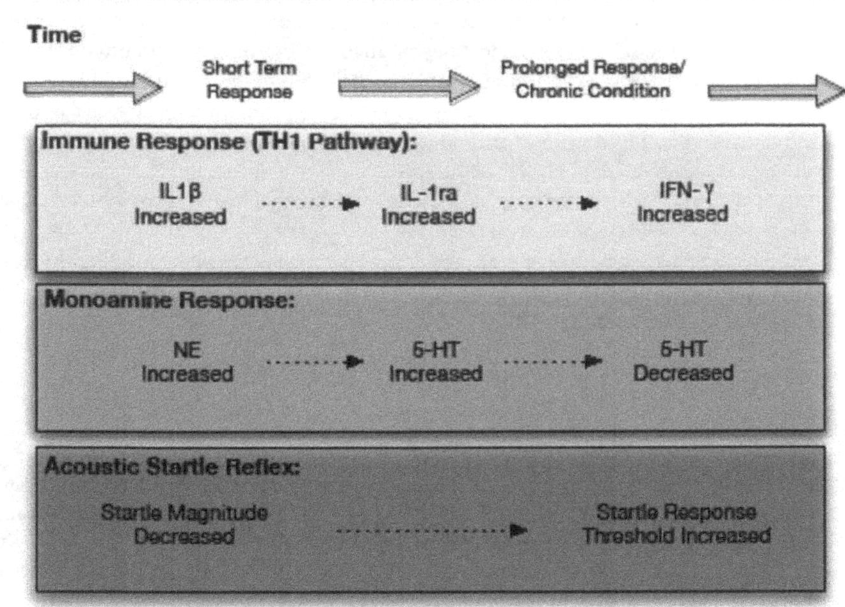

Figure 14. Based on the literature and the collected data from our laboratory, concerning the modulation of the ASR, we propose the following cascade of events may occur as a result of stressor exposure in our female rat model. First, the acute-phase (pro-inflammatory) response causes a transient reduction in startle responsivity (magnitude) that appears to last as long as IL-1 continues to be elevated above the levels of circulating IL-1ra. IL-1ra serves to normalize the response; thus, when the levels of IL-1ra are elevated to a sufficient degree, it causes an increase in ASR sensitivity (a rebound effect). However, in the cases where the stressor exposure is prolonged and/or severe enough to engage a downstream Th-1 response (i.e. increase IFN-γ signaling), then a reduction in ASR sensitivity occurs, whereby the sensory threshold for eliciting the response is increased. This could cause a chronic condition where ASRs are "blunted" in people with conditions ranging from PTSD to MDD to BPD.

The ASR could have a potential use as a functional index of abnormal peripheral immune functioning; thus, if the ASR is suppressed, it may represent an elevated level of pro-inflammatory or Th1 signaling in the patient. This could be of great importance from a therapeutic standpoint when one considers the suppressive effects of IL-1 upon sexual motivation in female rats are attenuated by indomethacin and ibuprofen [127]. Although blocking prostaglandin synthesis [128] or knocking-out the prostaglandin EP2 receptor does not change startle reactivity [129], prostaglandin EP1 knock-out mice do exhibit higher startle magnitudes compared to their wild-type control strain [130]. This suggests that EP1 receptors are in a position to serve as neuroimmune mechanisms to inhibit startle responsivity as well. Still, beyond the possible pharmacological implications, blunted reactivity to stimuli can have profound effects on other neural processes as well, and may explain some of the other symptoms associated with anxiety, MDD, or BPD. For instance, when the same dose of IL-1β, sufficient to blunt startle responsivity in female SD and Lewis rats, is administered to female SD rats prior to a simple associative learning procedure the rate of learning is slowed. This effect is attributed to a reduction in the neural representation of the unconditional reflexive response (i.e. the response is weaker), causing less optimal neural representation of the behavioral response to the predictive, conditional stimulus [131]. The implication is that associative learning may be impaired by either acute or chronic elevations in pro-inflammatory or Th1 cytokines. Interestingly, this pattern of effect is not observed in male rats, at these low to moderate dosages of IL-1β; in fact, these learning processes are facilitated [132, 133]. Thus, the ASR can serve as a tool to better understand the blunting of sensory reactivity, but may also have implications for more complex associative learning processes as well. In Figure 14, we present our theory as to how the ASR may be changed over time as a function of neuroimmune interactions between peripheral cytokine signaling (specifically the acute pro-inflammatory response and the downstream Th-1 response) and brain monoamines.

7. Conclusions

The evidence accumulated from these experiments favors a pro-inflammatory mechanism, over a HPA-axis glucocorticoid mechanism, as the necessary pathway that ultimately leads to the suppression of startle reactivity following stressor exposure. This finding adds to the ever-growing evidence that peripheral immune signaling has a significant role in influencing how the nervous systems functions. In this particular case, we have illustrated how a simple behavioral reflex can be dampened by pro-inflammatory signals, in the absence of any physical injury. This shows abnormal levels of peripheral immune signaling could lead to perceived symptoms reported by patients with PTSD, MDD, or BPD.

Biological differences in how different animals respond to stressor may reflect vulnerability factors for experiencing different symptoms associated with stress-related disorders, such as PTSD, MDD, and BPD. Thus, differences observed in the literature concerning startle reactivity in female PTSD patients (e.g. [18, 19]) could be due to the types of stressor exposure or individual differences in biological responses. In addition, one cannot rule-out the role of coping mechanisms. In fact, one could hypothesize that the suppression of startle is an evolutionary selected response that keeps individuals within a species from continuing to fight a "losing battle". If this were the case, then it would be logical for the immune system to play a role in that trigger-mechanism and not the HPA-axis. The HPA-axis is designed to maintain the fight-or-flight response [134], which would be in opposition to a behavioral suppression coping response. Others have proposed females are particularly selected to engage in alternative coping strategies that are in opposition to the fight-or-flight response [135], and one possibility is that signal reception of the peripheral immune response by the central nervous system is an early point of diversion in stress coping strategies between males and females. This could provide inherent propensities to respond differently, but, at the same time, could be modified by experience. Such propensities could translate into vulnerability factors for abnormal behaviors where that response becomes, potentially, maladaptive.

It is well documented that more women experience anxiety disorders and affective disorders, and there is a significant degree of comorbidity across these disorders – especially as cases become more severe [136]. There are many potential reasons for the higher rates reported in women. For instance, some have recently suggested there is a link between ovarian hormones and the occurrence of specific peptide isoforms that modulate stress responsiveness and fear conditioning [137]. The data presented here provide another example of how ovarian hormones can influence physiological processes associated with stress responsiveness. The role of progesterone in this immune model of startle suppression is particularly intriguing since progesterone can amplify the pro-inflammatory response through macrophage migration inhibitory factor [138]. This endocrine influence could, potentially, cause more Th1 signaling to occur, which, we hypothesize leads to an increase in IL-1β, causing more Th1 signaling to occur, eventually leading to an increase in IFN-γ release and subsequent reductions in sensitivity to auditory stimuli. If that same individual has central nervous system vulnerabilities, such as a particular peptide isoform, then, in addition to an apparent blunted startle response, the patient may also be exhibiting flashbacks due to enhanced neural processing of fear-associated memory. Thus, female vulnerability for anxiety and depression symptoms can be seen as a product of multiple mechanisms that modulate the female physiology and behavior in a manner that, at times, may even be counter to fight-or-flight, but, nonetheless lead to changes in nervous system functioning, causing the expression of a particular set of behavioral symptoms.

There is a growing literature pointing towards a complex interaction between the central nervous system and the peripheral immune system that underlies anxiety or affective disorder vulnerability and/or the presence of acute symptoms [139-143]. The utility of being able to use species-common measures, such as the startle response, has been advantageous to researchers in aiding them to understand how the brain functions under normal and abnormal conditions. Here we illustrate how such measures can be applied to the understanding of psychoneuroimmune interaction as they pertain to the influence of the peripheral immune system upon the brain and behavior. As we gain a greater understanding of the signaling cascades in the peripheral immune system, delineating how those signals affect the brain will continue to be important for our future understanding of the etiology of mental illnesses.

Acknowledgements

This research was supported by a U.S. Department of Veterans Affairs Merit Review research program to KDB and program support through the UMDNJ – Stress & Motivated Behavior Institute. The described experimentation was conducted with approval by the VANJHCS Institutional Animal Care and Use and Research and Development Committees, in accordance with the NIH Guide for the Care and Use of Animals. The authors want to thank Toni Marie Dispenziere, Tracey Longo, Ian Smith, and Paul William Ong for their technical assistance in conducting the experiments. Some of the described work was included in the undergraduate honors thesis of Mr. Ong. The authors also thank Dr. Victoria Luine for the use of the laboratory in the processing and measurement of the brain monoamine data.

Author details

Kevin D. Beck[1,2] and Jennifer E. Catuzzi[1,3]

1 Neurobehavioral Research Laboratory, Veteran Affairs New Jersey Health Care System, East Orange, NJ, USA

2 Stress & Motivated Behavior Institute, Department of Neurology & Neurosciences, University of Medicine & Dentistry of New Jersey – New Jersey Medical School, Newark, NJ, USA

3 University of Medicine & Dentistry of New Jersey – Graduate School of Biomedical Sciences, Newark, NJ, USA

References

[1] Davis M, Gendelman DS, Tischler MD, Gendelman PM. A primary acoustic startle circuit: lesion and stimulation studies. J Neurosci 1982 Jun;2(6):791-805.

[2] Davis M, Walker DL, Lee Y. Amygdala and bed nucleus of the stria terminalis: differential roles in fear and anxiety measured with the acoustic startle reflex. Philos Trans R Soc Lond B Biol Sci 1997 Nov 29;352(1362):1675-87.

[3] Davis M, Shi C. The extended amygdala: are the central nucleus of the amygdala and the bed nucleus of the stria terminalis differentially involved in fear versus anxiety? Ann N Y Acad Sci 1999 Jun 29;877:281-91.

[4] Walker DL, Toufexis DJ, Davis M. Role of the bed nucleus of the stria terminalis versus the amygdala in fear, stress, and anxiety. Eur J Pharmacol 2003 Feb 28;463(1-3): 199-216.

[5] Hitchcock J, Davis M. Lesions of the amygdala, but not of the cerebellum or red nucleus, block conditioned fear as measured with the potentiated startle paradigm. Behav Neurosci 1986 Feb;100(1):11-22.

[6] Falls WA, Davis M. Lesions of the central nucleus of the amygdala block conditioned excitation, but not conditioned inhibition of fear as measured with the fear-potentiated startle effect. Behav Neurosci 1995 Jun;109(3):379-87.

[7] Koch M, Kungel M, Herbert H. Cholinergic neurons in the pedunculopontine tegmental nucleus are involved in the mediation of prepulse inhibition of the acoustic startle response in the rat. Exp Brain Res 1993;97(1):71-82.

[8] Swerdlow NR, Geyer MA. Prepulse inhibition of acoustic startle in rats after lesions of the pedunculopontine tegmental nucleus. Behav Neurosci 1993 Feb;107(1):104-17.

[9] Koch M. The neurobiology of startle. Prog Neurobiol 1999 Oct;59(2):107-28.

[10] Koch M, Fendt M, Kretschmer BD. Role of the substantia nigra pars reticulata in sensorimotor gating, measured by prepulse inhibition of startle in rats. Behav Brain Res 2000 Dec 20;117(1-2):153-62.

[11] Morgan CA, III, Grillon C, Southwick SM, Davis M, Charney DS. Exaggerated acoustic startle reflex in Gulf War veterans with posttraumatic stress disorder. Am J Psychiatry 1996 Jan;153(1):64-8.

[12] Butler RW, Braff DL, Rausch JL, Jenkins MA, Sprock J, Geyer MA. Physiological evidence of exaggerated startle response in a subgroup of Vietnam veterans with combat-related PTSD. Am J Psychiatry 1990 Oct;147(10):1308-12.

[13] Grillon C, Morgan CA, III, Davis M, Southwick SM. Effect of darkness on acoustic startle in Vietnam veterans with PTSD. Am J Psychiatry 1998 Jun;155(6):812-7.

[14] Orr SP, Metzger LJ, Pitman RK. Psychophysiology of post-traumatic stress disorder. Psychiatric Clinics of North America 2002;25(2):271-93.

[15] American Psychiatric Association. Diagnostic and Statistical Manual of Mental Disorders. 4th-TR ed. Washington, DC: American Psychiatric Association; 2000.

[16] Grillon C, Baas J. A review of the modulation of the startle reflex by affective states and its application in psychiatry. Clin Neurophysiol 2003 Sep;114(9):1557-79.

[17] Ornitz EM, Pynoos RS. Startle modulation in children with posttraumatic stress disorder. Am J Psychiatry 1989 Jul;146(7):866-70.

[18] Medina AM, Mejia VY, Schell AM, Dawson ME, Margolin G. Startle reactivity and PTSD symptoms in a community sample of women. Psychiatry Res 2001 Mar 25;101(2):157-69.

[19] Fullerton CS, Ursano RJ, Epstein RS, Crowley B, Vance K, Kao TC, et al. Gender differences in posttraumatic stress disorder after motor vehicle accidents. Am J Psychiatry 2001 Sep;158(9):1486-91.

[20] Griffin MG. A prospective assessment of auditory startle alterations in rape and physical assault survivors. J Trauma Stress 2008 Feb;21(1):91-9.

[21] Morgan CA, III, Grillon C, Lubin H, Southwick SM. Startle reflex abnormalities in women with sexual assault-related posttraumatic stress disorder. Am J Psychiatry 1997 Aug;154(8):1076-80.

[22] Allen NB, Trinder J, Brennan C. Affective startle modulation in clinical depression: preliminary findings. Biol Psychiatry 1999 Aug 15;46(4):542-50.

[23] Forbes EE, Miller A, Cohn JF, Fox NA, Kovacs M. Affect-modulated startle in adults with childhood-onset depression: relations to bipolar course and number of lifetime depressive episodes. Psychiatry Res 2005 Mar 30;134(1):11-25.

[24] Bowers D, Miller K, Mikos A, Kirsch-Darrow L, Springer U, Fernandez H, et al. Startling facts about emotion in Parkinson's disease: blunted reactivity to aversive stimuli. Brain 2006 Dec;129(Pt 12):3356-65.

[25] Sloan DM, Sandt AR. Depressed mood and emotional responding. Biol Psychol 2010 May;84(2):368-74.

[26] Dichter GS, Tomarken AJ. The chronometry of affective startle modulation in unipolar depression. J Abnorm Psychol 2008 Feb;117(1):1-15.

[27] Giakoumaki SG, Bitsios P, Frangou S, Roussos P, Aasen I, Galea A, et al. Low baseline startle and deficient affective startle modulation in remitted bipolar disorder patients and their unaffected siblings. Psychophysiology 2010 Jul 1;47(4):659-68.

[28] Carroll CA, Vohs JL, O'donnell BF, Shekhar A, Hetrick WP. Sensorimotor gating in manic and mixed episode bipolar disorder. Bipolar Disord 2007 May;9(3):221-9.

[29] Conti LH, Printz MP. Rat strain-dependent effects of repeated stress on the acoustic startle response. Behav Brain Res 2003 Sep 15;144(1-2):11-8.

[30] Beck KD, Brennan FX, Servatius RJ. Effects of stress on nonassociative learning processes in male and female rats. Integr Physiol Behav Sci 2002 Apr;37(2):128-39.

[31] Beck KD, Servatius RJ. Stress-induced reductions of sensory reactivity in female rats depend on ovarian hormones and the application of a painful stressor. Horm Behav 2005 May;47(5):532-9.

[32] Beck KD, Jiao X, Cominski TP, Servatius RJ. Estrus cycle stage modifies the presentation of stress-induced startle suppression in female Sprague-Dawley rats. Physiol Behav 2008 Mar 18;93(4-5):1019-23.

[33] Adamec R, Strasser K, Blundell J, Burton P, McKay DW. Protein synthesis and the mechanisms of lasting change in anxiety induced by severe stress. Behav Brain Res 2006 Feb 28;167(2):270-86.

[34] Beck KD, Servatius RJ. Interleukin-1beta as a mechanism for stress-induced startle suppression in females. Ann N Y Acad Sci 2006 Jul;1071:534-7.

[35] Lockey AJ, Kavaliers M, Ossenkopp KP. Lipopolysaccharide produces dose-dependent reductions of the acoustic startle response without impairing prepulse inhibition in male rats. Brain Behav Immun 2008 Aug 3.

[36] Gonzales M, Garrett C, Chapman CD, Dess NK. Stress-induced attenuation of acoustic startle in low-saccharin-consuming rats. Biol Psychol 2008 Oct;79(2):193-9.

[37] Walker DL, Davis M. Anxiogenic effects of high illumination levels assessed with the acoustic startle response in rats. Biol Psychiatry 1997 Sep 15;42(6):461-71.

[38] Lee Y, Schulkin J, Davis M. Effect of corticosterone on the enhancement of the acoustic startle reflex by corticotropin releasing factor (CRF). Brain Res 1994 Dec 12;666(1): 93-8.

[39] Besedovsky H, del RA, Sorkin E, Dinarello CA. Immunoregulatory feedback between interleukin-1 and glucocorticoid hormones. Science 1986 Aug 8;233(4764):652-4.

[40] Sapolsky R, Rivier C, Yamamoto G, Plotsky P, Vale W. Interleukin-1 stimulates the secretion of hypothalamic corticotropin-releasing factor. Science 1987 Oct 23;238(4826):522-4.

[41] Rivier C, Vale W. In the rat, interleukin-1 alpha acts at the level of the brain and the gonads to interfere with gonadotropin and sex steroid secretion. Endocrinology 1989 May;124(5):2105-9.

[42] Turnbull AV, Rivier C. Regulation of the HPA axis by cytokines. Brain Behav Immun 1995 Dec;9(4):253-75.

[43] Schotanus K, Tilders FJ, Berkenbosch F. Human recombinant interleukin-1 receptor antagonist prevents adrenocorticotropin, but not interleukin-6 responses to bacterial endotoxin in rats. Endocrinology 1993 Dec;133(6):2461-8.

[44] Hosoi T, Okuma Y, Nomura Y. Electrical stimulation of afferent vagus nerve induces IL-1beta expression in the brain and activates HPA axis. Am J Physiol Regul Integr Comp Physiol 2000 Jul;279(1):R141-R147.

[45] Dhabhar FS, McEwen BS, Spencer RL. Stress response, adrenal steroid receptor levels and corticosteroid-binding globulin levels--a comparison between Sprague-Dawley, Fischer 344 and Lewis rats. Brain Res 1993 Jul 9;616(1-2):89-98.

[46] Klenerova V, Sida P, Hynie S, Jurcovicova J. Rat strain differences in responses of plasma prolactin and PRL mRNA expression after acute amphetamine treatment or restraint stress. Cell Mol Neurobiol 2001 Feb;21(1):91-100.

[47] Kusnecov AW, Shurin MR, Armfield A, Litz J, Wood P, Zhou D, et al. Suppression of lymphocyte mitogenesis in different rat strains exposed to footshock during early diurnal and nocturnal time periods. Psychoneuroendocrinology 1995;20(8):821-35.

[48] Zhu J, Zou LP, Bakhiet M, Mix E. Resistance and susceptibility to experimental autoimmune neuritis in Sprague-Dawley and Lewis rats correlate with different levels of autoreactive T and B cell responses to myelin antigens. J Neurosci Res 1998 Nov 1;54(3):373-81.

[49] Zhu J, Zou LP, Bakhiet M, Mix E. Resistance and susceptibility to experimental autoimmune neuritis in Sprague-Dawley and Lewis rats correlate with different levels of autoreactive T and B cell responses to myelin antigens. J Neurosci Res 1998 Nov 1;54(3):373-81.

[50] Redei E, Pare WP, Aird F, Kluczynski J. Strain differences in hypothalamic-pituitary-adrenal activity and stress ulcer. Am J Physiol 1994 Feb;266(2 Pt 2):R353-R360.

[51] Armario A, Gavalda A, Marti J. Comparison of the behavioural and endocrine response to forced swimming stress in five inbred strains of rats. Psychoneuroendocrinology 1995;20(8):879-90.

[52] Pardon MC, Gould GG, Garcia A, Phillips L, Cook MC, Miller SA, et al. Stress reactivity of the brain noradrenergic system in three rat strains differing in their neuroendocrine and behavioral responses to stress: implications for susceptibility to stress-related neuropsychiatric disorders. Neuroscience 2002;115(1):229-42.

[53] Watkins LR, Maier SF. Implications of immune-to-brain communication for sickness and pain. Proc Natl Acad Sci U S A 1999 Jul 6;96(14):7710-3.

[54] Dantzer R. Cytokine-induced sickness behavior: where do we stand? Brain Behav Immun 2001 Mar;15(1):7-24.

[55] Schmidt ED, Janszen AW, Wouterlood FG, Tilders FJ. Interleukin-1-induced long-lasting changes in hypothalamic corticotropin-releasing hormone (CRH)--neurons and hyperresponsiveness of the hypothalamus-pituitary-adrenal axis. J Neurosci 1995 Nov;15(11):7417-26.

[56] Schmidt ED, Schoffelmeer AN, De Vries TJ, Wardeh G, Dogterom G, Bol JG, et al. A single administration of interleukin-1 or amphetamine induces long-lasting increases in evoked noradrenaline release in the hypothalamus and sensitization of ACTH and corticosterone responses in rats. Eur J Neurosci 2001 May;13(10):1923-30.

[57] Fendt M, Li L, Yeomans JS. Brain stem circuits mediating prepulse inhibition of the startle reflex. Psychopharmacology (Berl) 2001 Jul;156(2-3):216-24.

[58] Semba K, Fibiger HC. Afferent connections of the laterodorsal and the pedunculopontine tegmental nuclei in the rat: a retro- and antero-grade transport and immunohistochemical study. J Comp Neurol 1992 Sep 15;323(3):387-410.

[59] Swerdlow NR, Geyer MA. Prepulse inhibition of acoustic startle in rats after lesions of the pedunculopontine tegmental nucleus. Behav Neurosci 1993 Feb;107(1):104-17.

[60] Koch M, Fendt M, Kretschmer BD. Role of the substantia nigra pars reticulata in sensorimotor gating, measured by prepulse inhibition of startle in rats. Behav Brain Res 2000 Dec 20;117(1-2):153-62.

[61] Bosch D, Schmid S. Activation of muscarinic cholinergic receptors inhibits giant neurones in the caudal pontine reticular nucleus. Eur J Neurosci 2006 Oct;24(7):1967-75.

[62] Koch M, Fendt M, Kretschmer BD. Role of the substantia nigra pars reticulata in sensorimotor gating, measured by prepulse inhibition of startle in rats. Behav Brain Res 2000 Dec 20;117(1-2):153-62.

[63] Lee Y, Davis M. Role of the septum in the excitatory effect of corticotropin-releasing hormone on the acoustic startle reflex. J Neurosci 1997 Aug 15;17(16):6424-33.

[64] Adams LM, Geyer MA. Effects of 6-hydroxydopamine lesions of locus coeruleus on startle in rats. Psychopharmacology (Berl) 1981;73(4):394-8.

[65] Simerly RB, Chang C, Muramatsu M, Swanson LW. Distribution of androgen and estrogen receptor mRNA-containing cells in the rat brain: an in situ hybridization study. J Comp Neurol 1990 Apr 1;294(1):76-95.

[66] Becker JB. Direct effect of 17 beta-estradiol on striatum: sex differences in dopamine release. Synapse 1990;5(2):157-64.

[67] Woolley CS, McEwen BS. Estradiol mediates fluctuation in hippocampal synapse density during the estrous cycle in the adult rat. J Neurosci 1992 Jul;12(7):2549-54.

[68] Koch M. Sensorimotor gating changes across the estrous cycle in female rats. Physiol Behav 1998 Jul;64(5):625-8.

[69] Gogos A, Van den BM. Estrogen and progesterone prevent disruption of prepulse inhibition by the serotonin-1A receptor agonist 8-hydroxy-2-dipropylaminotetralin. J Pharmacol Exp Ther 2004 Apr;309(1):267-74.

[70] Beck KD, McLaughlin J, Bergen MT, Cominski TP, Moldow RL, Servatius RJ. Facilitated acquisition of the classically conditioned eyeblink response in women taking oral contraceptives. Behav Pharmacol 2008 Dec;19(8):821-8.

[71] Toufexis DJ, Davis C, Hammond A, Davis M. Progesterone attenuates corticotropin-releasing factor-enhanced but not fear-potentiated startle via the activity of its neuroactive metabolite, allopregnanolone. J Neurosci 2004 Nov 10;24(45):10280-7.

[72] Lee Y, Davis M. Role of the hippocampus, the bed nucleus of the stria terminalis, and the amygdala in the excitatory effect of corticotropin-releasing hormone on the acoustic startle reflex. J Neurosci 1997 Aug 15;17(16):6434-46.

[73] Davis M, Walker DL, Lee Y. Roles of the amygdala and bed nucleus of the stria terminalis in fear and anxiety measured with the acoustic startle reflex. Possible relevance to PTSD. Ann N Y Acad Sci 1997 Jun 21;821:305-31.

[74] Sahuque LL, Kullberg EF, Mcgeehan AJ, Kinder JR, Hicks MP, Blanton MG, et al. Anxiogenic and aversive effects of corticotropin-releasing factor (CRF) in the bed nucleus of the stria terminalis in the rat: role of CRF receptor subtypes. Psychopharmacology (Berl) 2006 May;186(1):122-32.

[75] Walker D, Yang Y, Ratti E, Corsi M, Trist D, Davis M. Differential effects of the CRF-R1 antagonist GSK876008 on fear-potentiated, light- and CRF-enhanced startle suggest preferential involvement in sustained vs phasic threat responses. Neuropsychopharmacology 2009 May;34(6):1533-42.

[76] Lee Y, Lopez DE, Meloni EG, Davis M. A primary acoustic startle pathway: obligatory role of cochlear root neurons and the nucleus reticularis pontis caudalis. J Neurosci 1996 Jun 1;16(11):3775-89.

[77] Toufexis DJ, Davis C, Hammond A, Davis M. Progesterone attenuates corticotropin-releasing factor-enhanced but not fear-potentiated startle via the activity of its neuroactive metabolite, allopregnanolone. J Neurosci 2004 Nov 10;24(45):10280-7.

[78] Kash TL, Winder DG. Neuropeptide Y and corticotropin-releasing factor bi-directionally modulate inhibitory synaptic transmission in the bed nucleus of the stria terminalis. Neuropharmacology 2006 Oct;51(5):1013-22.

[79] Avitsur R, Donchin O, Barak O, Cohen E, Yirmiya R. Behavioral effects of interleukin-1 beta: modulation by gender, estrus cycle, and progesterone. Brain Behav Immun 1995 Sep;9(3):234-41.

[80] Toufexis DJ, Rochford J, Walker CD. Lactation-induced reduction in rats' acoustic startle is associated with changes in noradrenergic neurotransmission. Behav Neurosci 1999 Feb;113(1):176-84.

[81] Ericsson A, Kovacs KJ, Sawchenko PE. A functional anatomical analysis of central pathways subserving the effects of interleukin-1 on stress-related neuroendocrine neurons. J Neurosci 1994 Feb;14(2):897-913.

[82] Day HE, Akil H. Differential pattern of c-fos mRNA in rat brain following central and systemic administration of interleukin-1-beta: implications for mechanism of action. Neuroendocrinology 1996 Mar;63(3):207-18.

[83] Brebner K, Hayley S, Zacharko R, Merali Z, Anisman H. Synergistic effects of interleukin-1beta, interleukin-6, and tumor necrosis factor-alpha: central monoamine, corticosterone, and behavioral variations. Neuropsychopharmacology 2000 Jun ;22 (6): 566 -80 2000;22(6):566-80.

[84] Davis M, Cedarbaum JM, Aghajanian GK, Gendelman DS. Effects of clonidine on habituation and sensitization of acoustic startle in normal, decerebrate and locus coeruleus lesioned rats. Psychopharmacology (Berl) 1977 Mar 16;51(3):243-53.

[85] Albert DJ, Richmond SE. Reactivity and aggression in the rat: induction by alpha-adrenergic blocking agents injected ventral to anterior septum but not into lateral septum. J Comp Physiol Psychol 1977 Aug;91(4):886-96.

[86] Davis M. Neurochemical modulation of sensory-motor reactivity: acoustic and tactile startle reflexes. Neurosci Biobehav Rev 1980;4(2):241-63.

[87] Schulz B, Fendt M, Schnitzler HU. Clonidine injections into the lateral nucleus of the amygdala block acquisition and expression of fear-potentiated startle. Eur J Neurosci 2002 Jan;15(1):151-7.

[88] Davis M, Kehne JH, Commissaris RL. Antagonism of apomorphine-enhanced startle by alpha 1-adrenergic antagonists. Eur J Pharmacol 1985 Feb 5;108(3):233-41.

[89] Borsody MK, Weiss JM. Alteration of locus coeruleus neuronal activity by interleukin-1 and the involvement of endogenous corticotropin-releasing hormone. Neuroimmunomodulation 2002;10(2):101-21.

[90] Huang QJ, Jiang H, Hao XL, Minor TR. Brain IL-1 beta was involved in reserpine-induced behavioral depression in rats. Acta Pharmacol Sin 2004 Mar;25(3):293-6.

[91] Konsman JP, Parnet P, Dantzer R. Cytokine-induced sickness behaviour: mechanisms and implications. Trends Neurosci 2002 Mar;25(3):154-9.

[92] Konsman JP, Veeneman J, Combe C, Poole S, Luheshi GN, Dantzer R. Central nervous action of interleukin-1 mediates activation of limbic structures and behavioural depression in response to peripheral administration of bacterial lipopolysaccharide. European Journal of Neuroscience 2008 Dec;28(12):2499-510.

[93] Cunningham JT, Mifflin SW, Gould GG, Frazer A. Induction of c-Fos and DeltaFosB immunoreactivity in rat brain by Vagal nerve stimulation. Neuropsychopharmacology 2008 Jul;33(8):1884-95.

[94] Pacak K, McCarty R, Palkovits M, Kopin IJ, Goldstein DS. Effects of immobilization on in vivo release of norepinephrine in the bed nucleus of the stria terminalis in conscious rats. Brain Res 1995 Aug 7;688(1-2):242-6.

[95] Fendt M, Siegl S, Steiniger-Brach B. Noradrenaline transmission within the ventral bed nucleus of the stria terminalis is critical for fear behavior induced by trimethylthiazoline, a component of fox odor. J Neurosci 2005 Jun 22;25(25):5998-6004.

[96] Walker DL, Davis M. Double dissociation between the involvement of the bed nucleus of the stria terminalis and the central nucleus of the amygdala in startle increases produced by conditioned versus unconditioned fear. J Neurosci 1997 Dec 1;17(23): 9375-83.

[97] Koch M, Kungel M, Herbert H. Cholinergic neurons in the pedunculopontine tegmental nucleus are involved in the mediation of prepulse inhibition of the acoustic startle response in the rat. Exp Brain Res 1993;97(1):71-82.

[98] Swerdlow NR, Geyer MA. Prepulse inhibition of acoustic startle in rats after lesions of the pedunculopontine tegmental nucleus. Behav Neurosci 1993 Feb;107(1):104-17.

[99] Brebner K, Hayley S, Zacharko R, Merali Z, Anisman H. Synergistic effects of interleukin-1beta, interleukin-6, and tumor necrosis factor-alpha: central monoamine, corticosterone, and behavioral variations. Neuropsychopharmacology 2000 Jun;22(6): 566-80.

[100] Haywood SA, Simonian SX, van der Beek EM, Bicknell RJ, Herbison AE. Fluctuating estrogen and progesterone receptor expression in brainstem norepinephrine neurons through the rat estrous cycle. Endocrinology 1999 Jul;140(7):3255-63.

[101] Kataoka Y, Iijima N, Yano T, Kakihara K, Hayashi S, Hinuma S, et al. Gonadal regulation of PrRP mRNA expression in the nucleus tractus solitarius and ventral and lateral reticular nuclei of the rat. Brain Res Mol Brain Res 2001 Feb 19;87(1):42-7.

[102] Anderson ST, Kokay IC, Lang T, Grattan DR, Curlewis JD. Quantification of prolactin-releasing peptide (PrRP) mRNA expression in specific brain regions of the rat during the oestrous cycle and in lactation. Brain Res 2003 May 23;973(1):64-73.

[103] Morales T, Sawchenko PE. Brainstem prolactin-releasing peptide neurons are sensitive to stress and lactation. Neuroscience 2003;121(3):771-8.

[104] Xue B, Hay M. 17beta-estradiol inhibits excitatory amino acid-induced activity of neurons of the nucleus tractus solitarius. Brain Res 2003 Jun 20;976(1):41-52.

[105] Gaykema RP, Chen CC, Goehler LE. Organization of immune-responsive medullary projections to the bed nucleus of the stria terminalis, central amygdala, and paraventricular nucleus of the hypothalamus: evidence for parallel viscerosensory pathways in the rat brain. Brain Res 2007 Jan 26;1130(1):130-45.

[106] Mouihate A, Chen X, Pittman QJ. Interleukin-1beta fever in rats: gender difference and estrous cycle influence. Am J Physiol 1998 Nov;275(5 Pt 2):R1450-R1454.

[107] Mouihate A, Pittman QJ. Neuroimmune response to endogenous and exogenous pyrogens is differently modulated by sex steroids. Endocrinology 2003 Jun;144(6): 2454-60.

[108] Takahashi A, Ishimaru H, Ikarashi Y, Kishi E, Maruyama Y. Cholinergic input to the supraoptic nucleus increases Fos expression and body temperature in rats. Pflugers Arch 2001 Jun;442(3):451-8.

[109] Dunn AJ. Stress-related changes in cerebral catecholamine and indoleamine metabolism: lack of effect of adrenalectomy and corticosterone. J Neurochem 1988 Aug; 51(2):406-12.

[110] Swiergiel AH, Dunn AJ. Effects of interleukin-1beta and lipopolysaccharide on behavior of mice in the elevated plus-maze and open field tests. Pharmacol Biochem Behav 2007 Apr;86(4):651-9.

[111] Wieczorek M, Dunn AJ. Effect of subdiaphragmatic vagotomy on the noradrenergic and HPA axis activation induced by intraperitoneal interleukin-1 administration in rats. Brain Res 2006 Jul 26;1101(1):73-84.

[112] Wieczorek M, Swiergiel AH, Pournajafi-Nazarloo H, Dunn AJ. Physiological and behavioral responses to interleukin-1beta and LPS in vagotomized mice. Physiol Behav 2005 Jul 21;85(4):500-11.

[113] Swiergiel AH, Smagin GN, Johnson LJ, Dunn AJ. The role of cytokines in the behavioral responses to endotoxin and influenza virus infection in mice: effects of acute and chronic administration of the interleukin-1-receptor antagonist (IL-1ra). Brain Res 1997 Nov 21;776(1-2):96-104.

[114] Norra C, Becker S, Herpertz SC, Kunert HJ. Effects of experimental acute tryptophan depletion on acoustic startle response in females. Eur Arch Psychiatry Clin Neurosci 2008 Feb;258(1):1-9.

[115] Mann C, Croft RJ, Scholes KE, Dunne A, O'Neill BV, Leung S, et al. Differential effects of acute serotonin and dopamine depletion on prepulse inhibition and p50 suppression measures of sensorimotor and sensory gating in humans. Neuropsychopharmacology 2008 Jun;33(7):1653-66.

[116] Erhardt S, Schwieler L, Emanuelsson C, Geyer M. Endogenous kynurenic acid disrupts prepulse inhibition. Biol Psychiatry 2004 Aug 15;56(4):255-60.

[117] Woods AB, Page GG, O'Campo P, Pugh LC, Ford D, Campbell JC. The mediation effect of posttraumatic stress disorder symptoms on the relationship of intimate partner violence and IFN-gamma levels. Am J Community Psychol 2005 Sep;36(1-2): 159-75.

[118] Moffett JR, Namboodiri MA. Tryptophan and the immune response. Immunol Cell Biol 2003 Aug;81(4):247-65.

[119] Badovinac V, Mostarica-Stojkovic M, Dinarello CA, Stosic-Grujicic S. Interleukin-1 receptor antagonist suppresses experimental autoimmune encephalomyelitis (EAE) in rats by influencing the activation and proliferation of encephalitogenic cells. J Neuroimmunol 1998 May 1;85(1):87-95.

[120] Tohmi M, Tsuda N, Watanabe Y, Kakita A, Nawa H. Perinatal inflammatory cytokine challenge results in distinct neurobehavioral alterations in rats: implication in psychiatric disorders of developmental origin. Neurosci Res 2004 Sep;50(1):67-75.

[121] Petitto JM, McCarthy DB, Rinker CM, Huang Z, Getty T. Modulation of behavioral and neurochemical measures of forebrain dopamine function in mice by species-specific interleukin-2. J Neuroimmunol 1997 Mar;73(1-2):183-90.

[122] O'Brien SM, Scully P, Scott LV, Dinan TG. Cytokine profiles in bipolar affective disorder: focus on acutely ill patients. J Affect Disord 2006 Feb;90(2-3):263-7.

[123] Ortiz-Dominguez A, Hernandez ME, Berlanga C, Gutierrez-Mora D, Moreno J, Heinze G, et al. Immune variations in bipolar disorder: phasic differences. Bipolar Disord 2007 Sep;9(6):596-602.

[124] Su KP, Leu SJ, Yang YY, Shen WW, Chou YM, Tsai SY. Reduced production of interferon-gamma but not interleukin-10 in bipolar mania and subsequent remission. J Affect Disord 2002 Sep;71(1-3):205-9.

[125] Knijff EM, Breunis MN, Kupka RW, de Wit HJ, Ruwhof C, Akkerhuis GW, et al. An imbalance in the production of IL-1beta and IL-6 by monocytes of bipolar patients: restoration by lithium treatment. Bipolar Disord 2007 Nov;9(7):743-53.

[126] Boufidou F, Nikolaou C, Alevizos B, Liappas IA, Christodoulou GN. Cytokine production in bipolar affective disorder patients under lithium treatment. J Affect Disord 2004 Oct 15;82(2):309-13.

[127] Avitsur R, Weidenfeld J, Yirmiya R. Cytokines inhibit sexual behavior in female rats: II. Prostaglandins mediate the suppressive effects of interleukin-1beta. Brain Behav Immun 1999 Mar;13(1):33-45.

[128] Ross BM, Brooks RJ, Lee M, Kalasinsky KS, Vorce SP, Seeman M, et al. Cyclooxygenase inhibitor modulation of dopamine-related behaviours. Eur J Pharmacol 2002 Aug 23;450(2):141-51.

[129] Savonenko A, Munoz P, Melnikova T, Wang Q, Liang X, Breyer RM, et al. Impaired cognition, sensorimotor gating, and hippocampal long-term depression in mice lacking the prostaglandin E2 EP2 receptor. Exp Neurol 2009 May;217(1):63-73.

[130] Matsuoka Y, Furuyashiki T, Yamada K, Nagai T, Bito H, Tanaka Y, et al. Prostaglandin E receptor EP1 controls impulsive behavior under stress. Proc Natl Acad Sci U S A 2005 Nov 1;102(44):16066-71.

[131] Beck KD, Servatius RJ. Stress and cytokine effects on learning: what does sex have to do with it? Integr Physiol Behav Sci 2003 Jul;38(3):179-88.

[132] Servatius RJ, Beck KD. Facilitated acquisition of the classically conditioned eyeblink response in male rats after systemic IL-1beta. Integr Physiol Behav Sci 2003 Jul;38(3): 169-78.

[133] Brennan FX, Beck KD, Servatius RJ. Low doses of interleukin-1beta improve the leverpress avoidance performance of Sprague-Dawley rats. Neurobiol Learn Mem 2003 Sep;80(2):168-71.

[134] Selye H. Stress and disease. Science 1955;122:625-31.

[135] Taylor SE, Klein LC, Lewis BP, Gruenewald TL, Gurung RA, Updegraff JA. Biobehavioral responses to stress in females: tend-and-befriend, not fight-or-flight. Psychol Rev 2000 Jul;107(3):411-29.

[136] Kessler RC, McGonagle KA, Zhao S, Nelson CB, Hughes M, Eshleman S, et al. Lifetime and 12-month prevalence of DSM-III-R psychiatric disorders in the United States. Results from the National Comorbidity Survey. Arch Gen Psychiatry 1994 Jan; 51(1):8-19.

[137] Ressler KJ, Mercer KB, Bradley B, Jovanovic T, Mahan A, Kerley K, Norrholm SD, Kilaru V, Smith AK, Myers AJ, Ramirez M, Engel A, Hammack SE, Toufexis D, Braas

KM, Binder EB, May V. Post-traumatic stress disorder is associated with PACAP and the PAC1 receptor. Nature 2011 Feb; 470(7335): 492-497.

[138] Houdeau E, Moriez R, Leveque M, Salvador-Cartier C, Waget A, Leng L, Bueno L, Bucala R, Fioramonti J. Sex steroid regulation of macrophage migration inhibitory factor in normal and inflamed colon in the female rat. Gastroenterology 2007 Mar; 132(2): 982-93.

[139] Bauer ME, Wieck A, Lopes RP, Teixeira AL, Grassi-Oliveira R. Interplay between neuroimmunoendocrine systems during post-traumatic stress disorder: a minireview. Neuroimmunomodulation 2010;17(3):192-5.

[140] Pace TW, Heim CM. A short review on the psychoneuroimmunology of posttraumatic stress disorder: from risk factors to medical comorbidities. Brain Behav Immun 2011 Jan;25(1):6-13.

[141] Baker DG, Nievergelt CM, O'Connor DT. Biomarkers of PTSD: neuropeptides and immune signaling. Neuropharmacology 2012 Feb;62(2):663-73.

[142] Raison CL, Miller AH. Is depression an inflammatory disorder? Curr Psychiatry Rep 2011 Dec;13(6):467-75.

[143] Krishnadas R, Cavanagh J. Depression: an inflammatory illness? J Neurol Neurosurg Psychiatry 2012 May;83(5):495-502.

Chapter 7

Understanding and Treating Anxiety Disorders in Presence of Personality Disorder Diagnosis

Véronique Palardy, Ghassan El-Baalbaki,
Claude Bélanger and Catherine Fredette

Additional information is available at the end of the chapter

1. Introduction

The prevalence of personality disorders varies between 0.5% and 2.5% in the general population and it increases drastically in the clinical population [1, 2]. In a psychiatric population, about one half of all patients have pathological personality [3]. Following the multiaxial classification of the Diagnostic Manual of the American Psychiatric Association (DSM-IV-TR; [1]), Axis II personality disorders are defined as being stable, inflexible, and pervasive patterns of psychological experiences and behaviors that differ prominently from cultural expectations, and that lead to clinically significant distress or impairment in important areas of functioning. In the DSM-IV-TR, there are 10 distinct personality disorders organized into three clusters. Cluster "A" includes three personality disorders considered as odd or eccentric: paranoid, schizoid and schizotypal. Antisocial, borderline, narcissistic and histrionic personality disorders are grouped under Cluster "B", which is considered as the dramatic, emotional or erratic cluster. Finally, Cluster "C" comprises three anxious or fearful personality disorders: the avoidant personality disorder, the dependent personality disorder and the obsessive-compulsive personality disorder. In the next version of the DSM (DSM-V), the task force is proposing some major changes for Axis II and as per the may 1st 2012 online revision[4], the DSM-V will retain six personality disorder types : schizotypal, antisocial, borderline, narcissistic, avoidant and obsessive-compulsive.

The comorbidity between Axis I and Axis II disorders is much documented, and there are some voices in the scientific community that would even question whether or not the distinction between those two axis should be revisited [5-8]. Specifically, Axis II disorders have been found to be strongly associated with anxiety disorders [9, 10] and an increased prevalence of personality disorders has been found in patients with anxiety disorders [11, 12]. Personality disorders are associated to high social cost and mortality, such as crime, disability, underachievement, underemployment, increased need for medical care, institutionalization, suicide attempts, self-injurious behavior, family disruption, child abuse and neglect, poverty, and homelessness [12]. This underlies the importance of finding optimal treatment for this population, and understanding the mechanisms by which personality pathology interferes with other psychiatric disorders, such as anxiety disorders.

This chapter presents a comprehensive review of the literature on the co-occurrence of personality and anxiety disorders, and the treatment of the latter when comorbidity occurs. First, the influence of personality pathology on anxiety disorders in general is discussed, with no regard to specific anxiety disorders. Afterwards, the clinical features of each of the major anxiety disorders that are comorbid with personality disorders are examined separately. The influence of personality disorders on anxiety disorder symptomatology and on the course of illness is also discussed in terms of treatment. Emphasis will be on the outcome of cognitive and/or behavioral therapy, since its efficacy has been repeatedly established in the treatment of anxiety disorders. The influence of Axis II diagnosis on the outcome of pharmacological treatment of anxiety disorders is also briefly discussed. Major characteristics of the studies that are reviewed in the present chapter are presented in a table. Finally, future research questions on comorbidity of anxiety disorders in the presence of personality disorders are proposed.

2. Co-occurrence of personality disorders and anxiety disorders

From 36% to 76% of patients with anxiety disorders have been found to have a comorbid personality disorder diagnosis, with avoidant, dependent, obsessive-compulsive and paranoid being the most frequent [12]. Thus, anxiety disorders seem to be particularly associated with Cluster C personality disorders [13]. Personality disorders are known to be strongly associated with functional impairment [14], more severe psychopathology, and a decreased response to treatment [15]. When they coexist with anxiety disorders, the latter are characterized by chronicity and more functional impairment that when compared to anxiety disorders without Axis II comorbidity [11]. For example, in a study by Klass and colleagues [16], anxiety patients with comorbid personality disorders were three to four times more likely to have current dysthymia. Furthermore, patients with a personality disorder diagnosis were significantly more likely to present a past major depressive episode, and they received lower scores for current level of functioning, compared with a control group matched on primary anxiety diagnosis, sex, and age [16]. Moreover, the co-occurrence of personality disorders and anxiety disorders has been found to be associated with suicide. In one study, individuals with an anxiety disorder and antisocial personality disorder had more suicidal ideation and suicide attempts, in comparison to individuals with either disorder alone [17]. Finally, personality disorders were reported to have a negative prognostic impact on the naturalistic course of anxiety disorders. Ansell and colleagues [18] found that groups with higher rates of personality disorders generally showed a more complex and variable course of illness, which was characterized by frequent remissions and relapses, and the occurrence of new onsets of anxiety disorders over a 7-year period. Although, their sample was recruited among a treatment-seeking population, the purpose of this study was to investigate the naturalistic course of anxiety disorders. Thus, the treatment received was not controlled, and it was not considered in the analysis.

2.1. Etiology of comorbidity

It is likely that multiple mechanisms contribute to the co-occurrence of anxiety and personality disorders. One possible explanation is that Axis I and II disorders are etiologically independent and that apparent high rates of co-occurrence are simply due to high rates of each disorder[19]. However, Ruegg and Frances [12] argued that the high rates of co-occurrence found in several studies are due to sampling bias, since most studies have been made among treatment seeking populations. Given that treatment seeking generally correlates with higher symptomatology severity and with the presence of multiple comorbid disorders, it is likely that these samples overestimate the relationship between anxiety and personality disorders [12]. High rates of co-occurrence have also been explained by issues in assessing personality disorders among individuals with anxiety disorders. This refers to the "state versus trait" issue in comorbidity research [20]. Because mood state tend to color the perceptions, going through an episode of anxiety disorder may affect the patients' perception of their personality, which would result in a distorted report of the latter [19]. Thus, the presence of an Axis I disorder may result in a false positive diagnosis of personality disorder [12], which would lead to an overestimation of the prevalence of personality disorders among individuals with anxiety disorders. Several models have been proposed to explain the high rates of coexisting personality and anxiety disorders, and these are described in the following section.

First, it has been suggested that individuals with personality disorders are more *vulnerable* to develop comorbid disorders. Vulnerability models assume that the disorders are distinct but are causally related, such that the presence of one disorder increases the risk to develop the other [19]. For example, because of their interpersonal difficulties, individuals with personality disorders would be more prone to experience repeated, chronic and acute negative life events, such as failures and losses, which would then increase the risk to develop and/or maintain anxiety disorders [19]. Second, some studies have supported the hypothesis that personality disorder traits are risk factors for anxiety disorders. For example, schizotypal, antisocial, borderline, histrionic and dependent personality traits present in adolescence and early adulthood have been associated with higher risk of having an anxiety disorder by middle adulthood [21]. In one study [22], high narcissistic personality traits, measured one week after trauma, have been associated with an increased risk of developing posttraumatic stress disorder (PTSD) one month and four months after trauma, even when controlling for baseline anxiety disorders. However, Brandes and Bienvenu [23] mentioned that these findings do not consider possible causal mechanisms involved. For instance, personality disorder traits and anxiety disorders could share a common etiology, and personality disorder traits would only be earlier manifestations of these common causal influences [23]. Third, another model of comorbidity refers to overlapping criteria [24] and shared etiology [23]. Thus, characteristics of each disorder are viewed as manifestations of a common dimension of psychopathology, which would suggest that these disorders are not entirely distinct [19]. If they do share etiological factors, a shared genetic influence could be expected. Indeed, some results have supported the hypothesis of a common genetic base to anxiety and personality disorders. For instance, avoidant and dependent personality traits have been found to be more common in first-degree relatives of patients with panic disorder (PD) compared with relatives of control participants [25]. In another study, obsessive-compulsive traits were higher in first-degree relatives of patients with obsessive-compulsive disorder (OCD), compared with relatives of controls [26]. However, these findings could also be explained by environmental influences [23], since patients and their relatives could have lived in a similar environment. Fourth, the pathoplasty conceptualization emphasizes the influence of one condition on the presentation or course of the other, but does not assume a shared etiology [19]. Thus, one condition may have an additive effect on the other condition, or exacerbate the latter [27]. For example, avoidant personality disorder (AVPD) and panic disorder with agoraphobia (PDA) may have a pathoplastic relationship such that the presence of personality traits and anxious predispositions interact to promote the development of personality or anxiety disorders [18]. Finally, it has been suggested that personality disorder traits could be shaped by the experience of having an anxiety disorder in childhood or adolescence [23]. For example, current anxiety disorders among adolescents have been found to predict schizotypal, schizoid, borderline, avoidant, and dependent personality traits in early adulthood, even when controlling for other Axis I disorders during adolescence [28]. However, in this study, personality disorder traits have not been assessed during adolescence, so it cannot be concluded that they were subsequent to the development of anxiety disorders [23]. Results from Kasen and colleagues [29] gave additional support to this model. Indeed, the presence of an anxiety disorder in adolescence was found to predict an increased likelihood of having a paranoid personality disorder in young adulthood, when controlling for personality disorders in adolescence. Also, adolescents who reported anxiety symptoms that were increasing over time were more likely to have a paranoid personality disorder, or an OCPD in young adulthood [29]. The authors suggested that behaviors and thoughts associated with perfectionism and rigidity, which characterized OCPD, may develop to help control anxiety symptoms [29]. Yet, these findings still do not exclude the possibility that personality and anxiety disorders share a common etiology, although in this case, personality disorders would be the later manifestations [23]. Though all these models give interesting explanations to comorbidity of anxiety and personality disorders, they are not mutually exclusive and it is likely that more complex bio-psycho-social models are needed to explain the co-occurrence of these psychopathologies.

3. Influence of personality disorders on the outcome of treatment for anxiety disorders

Since patients with multiple psychopathologies are often excluded from treatment trials, comorbidity is often disregarded [30]. Thus, few controlled prospective studies have specifically examined the effect of comorbid personality disorders on the outcome of cognitive and behavioral treatment (CBT) for anxiety disorders. However, some studies have investigated this area of research, with interesting results.

The Reich and Green [31] review, based on studies of depressive and anxiety disorders, concluded that the presence of a personality disorder had a negative influence on the outcome of treatment for Axis I disorders. In fact, personality pathology was found to predict a negative outcome of treatment in practically all studies [31]. Another review [20], which covered empirical studies published between 1991 and 1993, yielded similar conclusions. However, with regard to anxiety disorders, only studies that investigated the outcome of treatment for PD or OCD were included in the two previous reviews. Although Reich confirmed the general conclusion that dysfunctional personality traits have a negative effect on the outcome of treatment for Axis I disorders in his latest review [32], he also reported that individuals with comorbid personality disorders show improvement of their anxiety disorder symptoms when treated for their anxiety disorder. However, in the Dreessen and Arntz [33] selective review, personality disorders were not found to predict negatively the outcome of psychological treatment for anxiety disorders. It was concluded that no specific personality disorder was consistently found to affect negatively treatment outcome of anxiety disorders, and that patients with a comorbid personality disorder were not more likely to select themselves out of treatment [33]. Finally, the authors reported that patients with a personality disorder generally do not respond less to cognitive and/or behavioral treatment for their anxiety disorder, compared to patients without a personality disorder. However, these authors also report in their review that personality disorders are found to have a negative effect on the outcome of pharmacological treatment for anxiety disorders.

4. Panic disorder with and without agoraphobia (PD/A)

Among panic patients, prevalence rates of comorbid personality disorders (mostly in the Cluster C) range from 37% to 60% [3, 34-42]. No study has yet established a clear link between a specific type of personality disorder and the diagnosis of PDA [43]. Some have reported a strong association of panic disorder with AVPD [35, 38], whereas others have found higher rates of obsessive-compulsive personality disorder (OCPD; [36, 44]). This being said, Mavissakalian, Hamann, and Jones [45] reported that personality disorders cannot be presumed to have specific etiological significance for PD, given that the personality disorder traits that are generally identified in PD patients are also present, and they are even more pronounced, in OCD patients.

4.1. Initial symptomatology and course of illness

Individuals with comorbid PD and personality disorders tend to present a higher clinical severity [3, 38, 44, 46] and a more chronic course of illness [41] than PD patients without a personality disorder. For instance, the presence of borderline personality disorder (BPD; [18]) or OCPD [47] was found to predict new onsets of PD, when no treatment is considered. In a study by Ozkan and Altindag [3], patients with comorbid PD and personality disorders had more severe anxiety, depression, and agoraphobic symptoms, onset was at younger age, and they had lower levels of functioning. On the other hand, Mellman and colleagues [37] found no significant differences in baseline clinical ratings, and on most measures of chronicity, severity and duration of PD in the presence of a personality disorder. In Ansell et al. study [18], the presence of an AVPD at baseline was even associated with a decreased likelihood of relapsing in their PDA.

In addition, comorbid personality disorders in PD patients have been associated with an increased risk of suicidal thoughts [44, 48] and suicide attempts [48]. In one study [49], all PD patients who had made serious suicide attempts had a comorbid personality disorder. A significant correlation between suicide attempts and comorbid Cluster B personality disorders was reported, particularly with BPD and histrionic personality disorder [49]. Other studies found a similar association of BPD with suicidal ideation [50] or suicide attempts [3] among PD patients. Also, paranoid personality disorder has been reported to predict suicide attempts, and AVPD to predict suicidal ideation among this population [3]. Moreover, it appears that personality disorder criteria do not necessarily need to be met to aggravate the severity of PD. Indeed, studies have found personality disorder traits to be associated with more baseline clinical disturbance among this population. For instance, PD patients with a greater number of personality disorder traits have been found to be more symptomatic on almost all measures of psychopathology [51].

4.2. Influence of personality pathology on the outcome of cognitive and/or behavioral treatment for panic disorder with and without agoraphobia

Studies examining the effect of personality disorders on the outcome of cognitive and/or behavioral therapy for PD have obtained conflicting results. However, as can be expected, many studies have found a negative impact of personality disorders on the outcome of treatment. Tyrer and colleagues [52] randomly assigned 181 patients with generalized anxiety disorder (GAD), PD, or dysthymia to three modalities of treatment: pharmacological treatment, cognitive therapy, or self–help. Their results indicated that the presence of a personality disorder did negatively influence the outcome of cognitive therapy and self–help at the 2-year follow-up test. Using the same sample to measure the effect of time on treatment outcome, Seivewright, Tyrer, and Johnson [53] found that the presence of a personality disorder was still associated with a negative prognostic indicator five years after cognitive therapy. Other studies also found a negative influence of personality disorders on the outcome of CBT [38] or behavioral treatment [54] for PD. Keijsers, Schaap, and Hoogduin [55] found that higher personality psychopathology, as measured by the revised version of the personality diagnostic questionnaire ((PDQ-R; [56]) scores, was related to higher levels of agoraphobic avoidance and higher frequency of panic attacks after behavioral treatment. Yet, the relationship was no longer significant after statistical adjustment for multiple tests [55]. Chambless and colleagues [57] examined the effects of secondary major depression, dysthymia, GAD, and AVPD on the outcome of a behavioral treatment, which mostly consisted of an exposure-based individual treatment, and a group psychotherapy that focused on interpersonal and intrapsychic problems that were believed to maintain their PDA. Their results indicated that AVPD predicted less improvement in the frequency of panic attacks at the 6-month follow-up. Finally, the influence of specific clusters of personality disorders on treatment outcome has been found to vary depending on whether personality pathology was assessed dimensionally or categorically. For example, the presence of a Cluster A diagnosis was the strongest predictor of CBT outcome when assessed categorically, whereas these Cluster A disorders were not associated with CBT outcome when assessed dimensionally [38].

In other studies, comorbid personality disorders have been found to have little or no impact on the outcome of cognitive and/or behavioral treatment for PD. Dreessen, Arntz, Luttels, and Sallaerts [58] results suggest that PD patients with and without personality disorders profit equally from CBT for their PD, although certain personality disorder traits were found to have some impact on treatment outcome. Indeed, OCPD traits were negatively related to treatment outcome, and borderline traits predicted better outcome, but this latter finding was only observed at the 6-month follow-up test. However, given that personality disorders were lumped together to obtain adequate sample sizes, the influence of individual personality disorders on the outcome of CBT for PD was not measured [58]. Black and colleagues [59] studied treatment response in 66 PD patients who had completed three weeks of treatment with cognitive therapy, pharmacotherapy, or placebo pharmacotherapy. Surprisingly, this study yielded different conclusions depending on the measurement method used to assess personality functioning. The presence of a personality disorder assessed by the Structured Interview for DSM-III-R Personality disorders (SIDP; Stangl et al., 1987] was not a predictor of treatment outcome at week four whereas the presence of a personality disorder assessed by a self-report questionnaire was a negative predictor of outcome in the groups receiving cognitive therapy or placebo [59]. In their selective review, Dreessen and Arntz [33] also examined the two previous studies, and the Chambless et al. [57] study. They concluded that personality disorders do not seem to significantly affect the outcome of cognitive and/or behavioral treatment for PD, but when personality disorders are examined separately, AVPD appears to be associated with a less favorable outcome in the long term, although it has no effect on immediate outcome [33]. To our knowledge, two other studies also concluded that patients with and without personality disorders seem to profit equally from CBT for their PDA [60, 61]. Hofmann and colleagues [62] found similar results. Indeed, personality disorder characteristics, as measured by the Wisconsin Personality Disorders Inventory (WISPI; [63]) were not found to predict outcome of CBT for PD. Finally, Kampman, Keijsers, Hoogduin, and Hendriks [64] examined whether Cluster C personality disorders predicted treatment response in a sample of 161 PD patients treated with CBT. Their results indicated that the presence of Cluster C personality disorders did not affect treatment outcome. These researchers [64] suggested that their results may be explained by the use of a self-report questionnaire to assess personality (PDQ-R), which is known to have high sensitivity, and moderate specificity [65].

4.3. Pharmacological treatment

The presence of a comorbid personality disorder has been found to be one of the most robust predictors of nonresponse to pharmacological treatment for PD [66]. For example, Marchesi and colleagues [67], in a study with 71 PD patients, found a negative effect of borderline personality traits on the outcome of selective serotonin reuptake inhibitor (SSRI) pharmacological treatment. In their study, Green and Curtis [35] measured the effect of personality disorders on the outcome of a pharmacological treatment (participants were treated with a tricyclic antidepressant or an anxiolytic) among 25 PD patients. There was a significant relationship between the presence of at least one personality disorder and relapse, and with regard to specific personality disorders, AVPD was associated with an increased likelihood of relapse. Reich [42] found a negative association between the outcome of pharmacological treatment (benzodiazepine molecules) and the presence of borderline, antisocial, histrionic, and narcissistic personality disorders. However, other studies [62, 68] did not find an influence of personality disorders on the outcome of pharmacological treatment for PD. The Tyrer et al. study [52] mentioned previously also found no influence of personality disorders on the outcome of pharmacological treatment for PD, which is inconsistent with conclusions drawn from Dreessen and Arntz review [33]. This is explained by the fact that the Tyrer et al. study [52] has not been reviewed by Dreessen and Arntz [33], given that it did not meet the "best-evidence criteria" needed to be included in the review. Indeed, the authors only reviewed the studies that met the two criteria that they believed would meet the best designed studies, which are a prospective design, and the use of a structured, or semi-structured, interview.

In some studies, treatment consisted of combined CBT and pharmacotherapy. In one study [69], comorbid personality disorders were associated with a delayed response to pharmacotherapy and behavioral treatment for PD, and the association was stronger for AVPD. In another study [70], 60 PD patients were treated with SSRIs and CBT, or with CBT only. Results indicated that treatment for patients without a personality disorder was significantly more effective with regard to general psychopathology, PD symptoms, and depression. However, there were no differences between groups on overall symptoms of anxiety, as measured by Hamilton Anxiety Scale and Beck Anxiety Inventory [70-72].

5. Obsessive-Compulsive Disorder (OCD)

Studies have found prevalence rates of comorbid personality disorders of 49% to 75% in patients with OCD, and personality disorders from Cluster C were found to be the most diagnosed [45, 73-77]. As can be expected, many studies have reported OCPD to be the most diagnosed among clinical samples of OCD patients [26, 73, 75, 78-82], with prevalence rates of 18% to 55% [75, 78, 80]. However, other studies have found much lower rates of OCPD among OCD patients (6% for Baer et al. [83]; 4% for Joffee, Swinson, & Regan [84]; 4% for Steketee [77]).

5.1. Initial symptomatology and course of illness

OCD patients with comorbid personality disorders do not seem to have more severe OCD symptoms compared to those without personality disorders [76, 77, 80]. Cavedini and colleagues [78] found no differences in the severity of OCD symptoms at baseline between OCD patients with and without OCPD. However, studies indicate more depressive and anxious symptoms, and more impairment in functioning before treatment in OCD patients with comorbid Axis II diagnosis [76, 81]. Bejerot and colleagues [73] found similar results. In their study, higher scores on all anxiety scales, and more functional impairment were reported for OCD individuals with comorbid personality disorders. In the Fricke et al. [80] study, the presence of a personality disorder was associated with more depressive symptoms and higher levels of functional impairment. In addition, the presence of an OCPD [18, 85] or an AVPD was found to predict new onsets of OCD, and the presence of a BPD diagnosis at baseline was associated with an increased likelihood of relapsing in OCD, when no treatment was considered [18].

5.2. Influence of personality pathology on the outcome of cognitive and/or behavioral treatment for OCD

Baer and Jenike [86] reviewed the presence of comorbid personality disorders in OCD patients and their influence on treatment outcome. They concluded that schizotypal personality disorder was the only one that predicted poorer outcome of treatment (behavioral or pharmacological) for OCD. Although this Axis II disorder is not particularly common among patients with OCD [26], schizotypal personality disorder and traits have been repeatedly related to poor response to behavioral treatment for OCD [87, 88]. Moritz and colleagues [89] suggest that it may be the positive schizotypal symptoms (e.g. unusual perceptual experiences, paranoid ideation, sensory irritation, magical beliefs) that predict poor treatment outcome. Impairment of learning [88] and difficulties to comply with treatment [90] have also been suggested to explain nonresponse to OCD treatment among individuals with a schizotypal personality disorder. Moreover, OCD patients with a schizotypal personality disorder may respond better to low-dose atypical neuroleptics and specialized CBT for schizotypal symptoms [89]. Other personality disorders have been associated with a less favorable outcome of CBT among OCD patients. In one study [91], OCD patients with any Cluster A or Cluster B personality disorder showed a poorer response to behavioral treatment or CBT at 12-month follow-up, compared with patients without these diagnoses.

Some studies have found no effect of personality disorders on the outcome of CBT for OCD. Dreessen and colleagues [79] studied 43 OCD patients who completed a behavioral or cognitive treatment, or a CBT. The presence of one or more personality disorders had no impact on the outcome of treatment. Indeed, patients with personality disorders did not differ in their improvement from patients without a personality disorder, and they dit not differ on their end-state functioning. Moreover, those who abandoned treatment did not differ from completers with regard to personality disorder characteristics. In another study [80], influence of personality disorders on the outcome of CBT has been compared for 24 OCD patients with comorbid personality disorders, and 31 without a personality disorder. Results indicated that both groups benefited equally from treatment, and were able to maintain their improvement at follow-up. Steketee [77] also found no association between personality disorders and the outcome of a behavioral treatment for OCD. However, the author suggested that an unsufficient statistical power might have explained that no differences in outcome were found between patients with and without a personality disorder [77]. Surprisingly, a positive impact of personality disorder traits on treatment outcome was found: patients with dependent or avoidant personality traits had improved significantly more on target symptoms at posttest. Yet, the improvement was not maintained during the follow-up period. No explanation was proposed for this unusual finding, and it should be carefully interpreted given the small sample size in this study (n=26).

5.3. Pharmacological treatment

The presence of a comorbid schizotypal personality disorder has also been associated with poorer outcome of pharmacological treatment [87, 90, 92], and of combined behavioral and pharmacological treatment [88] for OCD. In one study [93], the presence of schizotypal personality disorder, AVPD, or BPD, and the presence of any Cluster A diagnosis were associated with poorer outcome of a tricyclic antidepressant treatment (TCA) for OCD. Cavedini and colleagues [78] found a negative influence of OCPD on the outcome of a pharmacological treatment. Thus, poorer response to TCA or SSRI treatment was reported in OCD patients with OCPD than those without the comorbid Axis II diagnosis. However, one study [94] found no effect of personality disorders on the outcome of an SSRI medication for OCD. An association with outcome was only found for AVPD, which was associated with greater improvement on OCD symptoms.

6. Generalized Anxiety Disorder (GAD)

Studies have reported prevalence rates of personality disorders of 35% to 50% among patients with GAD [13, 95-98]. Compared with PD patients, GAD patients have been found to be more likely to have at least one personality disorder [13]. Similar to personality disorders, GAD seems to be more trait-like than state-like, since its symptoms are fairly continuous and lasting in time [13]. Thus, it has been suggested that personality disorders may be a more important factor in the development of GAD than they are for other anxiety disorders [13, 99]. Although GAD does not seem to have a strong association with a particular type of personality disorder [100], Dyck and colleagues [13] found AVPD to be the most prevalent (22%) in their sample of 122 GAD patients. Some correlations have also been found with obsessive-compulsive traits [101], OCPD [102], and dependent personality disorder [96].

6.1. Initial symtomatology and course of illness

There is an association between low social functioning and the presence of personality disorders among GAD population, although the relation seems to be specific to certain areas of functioning [103]. Indeed, results indicated no significant association between the presence of a personality disorder and functioning with mates, siblings, or functioning as a student. In addition, personality disorders were found to influence the naturalistic course of GAD. For instance, Ansell and colleagues [18] found that GAD patients with OCPD or BPD at baseline were more likely to have a GAD relapse, and those with OCPD were also more likely to have a new episode onset of GAD, compared with patients without these personality disorders. Also, schizotypal personality disorder was found to be the strongest predictor of chronicity, which was measured by the proportion of weeks spent in episode of GAD [18].

In another study [95], the presence of AVPD or dependent personality disorder explained the lower probability of remission from GAD.

6.2. Influence of personality pathology on the outcome of cognitive and/or behavioral treatment for GAD

Very few studies have examined the effect of personality disorders on the outcome of CBT for GAD. The lack of treatment studies with GAD patients may be partly explained by the fact that this anxiety disorder was not officially recognized as a primary diagnostic category until the appearance of the DSM-III-R [104]. However, Sanderson, Beck, and McGinn [97] examined the effect of personality disorders on the immediate outcome of a cognitive therapy for 22 patients with GAD. Although there were no significant differences in improvement and end-state functioning in patients with and without personality disorders, patients with a comorbid personality disorder were more likely to drop out of treatment [97]. In addition, the Tyrer et al. study [52] mentioned previously found a negative influence of personality disorders on the outcome of CBT for GAD.

6.3. Pharmacological treatment

To our knowledge, very few controlled prospective studies have examined the link between the presence of a personality disorder and the outcome of pharmacological treatment for GAD. Although they did find an influence of personality disorders on the outcome of CBT, Tyrer and colleagues [52] found no effect of personality disorders on the outcome of pharmacotherapy for GAD. One retrospective study [102] examined the effect of personality disorders on the outcome of a benzodiazepine drug treatment for GAD. The results indicated that chronic GAD patients were more likely to have Cluster B or C disorders than were remitted GAD patients. However, it is impossible to assume that outcome is due to the original drug treatment because participants had not been assessed immediately after treatment. In fact, participants were only interviewed 16 months after treatment, and during the follow-up period, they have had different types of treatment, pharmacological or psychological. Also, personality disorders were not assessed before treatment [102]. Thus, based on these results only, it cannot be concluded that personality disorders have a negative effect on the outcome of pharmacological treatment for GAD.

7. Social phobia

The rate of personality disorder diagnoses has been reported to be generally higher among social phobic patients than among patients with other Axis I conditions [13, 15]. Among anxiety disorder patients, some studies have also found the highest rates of personality disorders to be among patients with social phobia [16, 98]. The prevalence of personality disorders among social phobic patients ranges from 24% to 56% [105-107]. A strong association has been found between social phobia and AVPD [107-110]. Indeed, Dyck and colleagues [13] results indicated that individuals with social phobia were more than two times more likely to have an AVPD, compared with patients with PD or GAD. Overall, studies have reported 36% to 89% of comorbidity between AVPD and the generalized subtype of social phobia [13, 111-114]. In fact, questions have been raised about the validity of the existing categorical distinction between these two disorders [15, 23, 105]. Indeed, DSM-IV-TR criterion A for social phobia ("a marked and persistent fear of one or more social or performance situations in which the person is exposed to unfamiliar people or to possible scrutiny by others; the individual fears that he or she will act in a way (or show anxiety symptoms) that will be humiliating or embarrassing") overlaps with criterion four of AVPD ("the individual is preoccupied with being criticized or rejected in social situations"). In addition, DSM-IV-TR criterion D for social phobia ("the feared social or performance situations are avoided or else are endured with intense anxiety or distress") overlaps with criteria one ("avoids occupational activities that involve significant interpersonal contact, because of fears of criticism, disapproval, or rejection") and seven ("is unusually reluctant to take personal risks or to engage in any new activities because they may prove embarrassing") for AVPD. Furthermore, given that studies have found few cases of AVPD without generalized social phobia [115, 116], it has been suggested that AVPD could represent a subtype of more severe social phobia [15, 39]. In a review of literature on this subject, Widiger [116] concluded that there is no evidence indicating a clear demarcation between the two disorders, and that they appear to be a single disorder. Moreover, a recent twin study [117] found a common genetic vulnerability to women with AVPD and women with social phobia, which gives support to the hypothesis of a shared etiology. Even though the literature has focused on the association of social phobia with AVPD, other personality disorders have been found to be prevalent among social phobics. In their review, Johnson and Lydiard [15] reported OCPD and dependent personality disorder to be the second most prevalent among social phobics. Thus, social phobia seems to be particularly associated with Cluster C personality disorders.

7.1. Initial symptomatology and course of illness

In most studies, social phobic patients with comorbid personality disorders are reported to be more severely impaired before treatment. Mersch and colleagues [106] showed that social phobic patients with a comorbid personality disorder presented a more severe symptom pattern at baseline, with more irrational and negative thinking patterns, compared to those without a personality disorder. Moreover, two studies found more depressive symptoms for social phobic patients with personality disorders compared to those without an Axis II diagnosis [15, 107]. Herbert and colleagues [112] compared patients with generalized social phobia with and without AVPD, and found that patients with AVPD had more comorbid pathology, impairment in functioning, and reported higher levels of severity on all measures, including fear of negative evaluation, social avoidance and distress, depression and general psychopathology. Other studies have reported social phobic patients with a comorbid AVPD to have a more severe baseline symptomatology compared to those without an AVPD [111, 113]. In addition, the presence of a personality disorder, and more specifically an AVPD, has been associated with a decreased likelihood of remission from social phobia, when no treatment is considered [18, 95]. Patients with this comorbidity are also more likely to have a new episode onset of social phobia, in comparison to social phobics without an AVPD [18]. A comorbid AVPD was also found to be the strongest predictor of chronicity of social phobia [18]. Finally, the presence of a schizotypal personality disorder has been associated with an increased likelihood of social phobia relapse [18]. Given that it may be difficult to distinguish between long-standing social fears and Cluster A personality disorder symptoms, the latter finding could be explained by an erroneous assessment [115]. Thus, the social isolation would not be the result of a social anxiety, but rather a consequence of the paranoid thinking that generally characterizes an individual with a schizotypal personality disorder.

7.2. Influence of personality pathology on the outcome of cognitive and/or behavioral treatment for social phobia

Outcome studies have shown that there is no effect of personality disorders on the outcome of cognitive and/or behavioral treatment for social anxiety. For instance, a study [106] examining the outcome of two forms of treatment for social phobia, an exposure-based treatment or CBT, showed that patients with a comorbid personality disorder have been found to improve as much as those without a personality disorder. Another study [110] also indicated no differences on the outcome of a behavioral therapy with regard to the presence or absence of a comorbid personality disorder. Indeed, results indicated that patients with and without personality disorders improved at the same rate on social phobic avoidance, cognitions, and target situations that needed to be changed.

Because of its strong association with social phobia, many studies examined the specific effect of AVPD on the outcome of treatment. Feske and colleagues [111] examined its effect on the outcome of an exposure-based therapy for 48 patients with social phobia. Those with an AVPD improved less with regard to trait anxiety and self-esteem at posttest, but no differences in improvement rates were found with regard to depression, social adjustment and social phobic complaints. Although patients with an AVPD continued to have more severe symptomatology than those without AVPD at posttest and 3-month follow-up, both groups improved at the same rate during the follow-up period. However, the authors mentioned that interpretation of the follow-up data is difficult because of the additional uncontrolled treatments received during this period [111]. Other studies also reported no effect of AVPD on the outcome of cognitive and/or behavioral treatment for social phobia [110, 113, 118, 119]. Thus, evidence suggests no influence of AVPD on the outcome of CBT for social phobia.

To our knowledge, only one study [120] found a negative impact of personality disorders on the outcome of a cognitive and behavioral group treatment for social phobic patients. After treatment, patients without a personality disorder had improved significantly more on all outcome measures, except for the State-Trait Anxiety Inventory (STAI) and on the rating of avoidance of worst fear, for which there were no significant differences [120]. However, these results should be carefully interpreted, given that the effect sizes are very small for all of these outcome measures.

7.3. Pharmacological treatment

Very few studies have examined the impact of Axis II diagnosis on the outcome of pharmacological treatment for social phobia. To our knowledge, one study [121] has found a negative influence of personality disorders on the outcome of a pharmacological treatment for social phobia. In this study [121], long-term treatment with moclobemide (monoamine oxidase inhibitor; MAOI) was investigated among 101 social phobic patients. Treatment consisted of four years of moclobemide, with a drug-free period of at least one month, after the first two years. Dependent personality disorder and AVPD were diagnosed in 16% and 72% of patients, respectively. Results indicated that Axis II diagnosis predicted non-response to moclobemide.

8. Posttraumatic Stress Disorder (PTSD)

High rates of personality disorders have been found among individuals with PTSD [122-124]. Studies have reported comorbid Axis II diagnosis in 39% to 45% of PTSD patients [125, 126]. A strong association has been found between PTSD and BPD [127, 128]. For example, Zanarini and colleagues [129] results indicated that PTSD was significantly more diagnosed among BPD patients than among patients with other personality disorders. Also, in a sample of 34 male combat veterans with PTSD, BPD was the most common Axis II diagnosis, with a prevalence rate of 76% [123]. Shea and colleagues [124] also reported high rates of BPD [68%) among PTSD patients.

Given that past events of traumatic exposure are commonly reported by individuals with BPD [130], a history of trauma has been proposed to have a formative role in the development of BPD [131-133]. However, a strong association between the two disorders has not been found consistently across studies. In two other studies [126, 134], only 10% of PTSD patients had a comorbid BPD. Hembree and colleagues [126] suggested that these low rates might be explained by the exclusion of patients with current suicidal plans or intentions, and those with self-injurious behaviors from both studies. Since these characteristics are commonly present among individuals with BPD, this could have possibly led to the exclusion of a significant amount of BPD patients in those studies.

8.1. Initial symptomatology and course of illness

PTSD patients with comorbid personality disorders may experience a more severe course of illness than PTSD patients without personality disorders [135]. More specifically, Ansell and colleagues [18] found that PTSD patients with a schizotypal personality disorder at baseline were less likely to remit from PTSD than patients without a schizotypal diagnosis [18]. Surprisingly, their results also suggest that the presence of an OCPD is associated with a positive course of illness for PTSD. Indeed, patients with an OCPD at intake were less likely to have a PTSD relapse [18]. This could be explained by the fact that OCPD is characterized by perfectionism, meticulosity, rigidity, and extreme devotion to work and efficiency (DSM-IV-TR), which may lead to a good compliance with treatment. As mentioned previously, although Ansell and colleagues [18] investigated the naturalistic course of anxiety disorders, they recruited their sample among a treatment-seeking population. Even though no treatment was controlled in this study, the patients still received some form of treatment during the 7-year period of the study. Thus, OCPD patients, because of their possibly good compliance with treatment, might have respond better to treatment for their PTSD, which might have led to a decreased likelihood of relapse.

However, most studies have specifically measured the impact of BPD on pretreatment symptomatology of PTSD patients. For instance, Axis I diagnoses were found to be more prevalent among individuals with coexisting PTSD and BPD, in comparison to individuals with PTSD alone [128]. A comorbid BPD diagnosis has also been associated with greater psychosocial impairment [128], and higher general distress [127, 136]. Moreover, studies have reported greater suicide proneness [128] among PTSD individuals with comorbid BPD, compared with PTSD individuals without BPD. Also, PTSD patients with comorbid BPD were reported to be more severely disturbed with regard to PTSD symptoms [127], although other studies did not find such differences between PTSD patients with and without comorbid BPD [136, 137]. Feeny and colleagues [134] also found no group differences on measures of anxiety, depression, and social functioning with regard to the presence or absence of partial, or complete BPD diagnosis.

8.2. Influence of personality pathology on the outcome of cognitive and/or behavioral treatment for posttraumatic stress disorder

As for other anxiety disorders, studies have yielded conflicting findings with regard to the effect of Axis II diagnosis on the outcome of CBT for PTSD. In the Hembree et al. [126] study, there were no significant differences between women with and without personality disorders on the prevalence of PTSD at the end of CBT or prolonged exposure. However, significantly more participants without a personality disorder (76%) achieved good end-state functioning status than participants with a personality disorder (41%). However, the group with personality disorders had higher scores on measures of PTSD symptoms, anxiety, and depression at pretreatment compared to the group without personality disorders, which could explain that this group was less likely to achieve a good end-state functioning [126]. In their retrospective study, Feeny and colleagues [134] examined the effect of borderline personality characteristics on the outcome of cognitive and/or behavioral therapy among 72 women with PTSD. Their results indicated that the group without borderline personality characteristics (described as having no significant BPD symptoms) had achieved a better end-state functioning at posttest, although this result was not obtained at the 3-month follow-up. However, there were no differences between groups on PTSD status, and outcome measures at posttest and follow-up [134].

In one study [138] examining predictors of outcome for PTSD patients treated with an exposure-based treatment, personality disorders were not found to predict treatment outcome, or premature dropout. In their retrospective study, Clarke and colleagues [127] found similar results with regard to borderline personality characteristics. Their results indicated that PTSD women with higher rates of borderline personality characteristics benefited as much from CBT, and that they were not more likely to drop out of treatment. To our knowledge, no study has examined the influence of personality disorders on the outcome of pharmacological treatment for PTSD.

Authors	Year	Participants	Treatment	Influence of personality disorders on outcome	Other results
Tyrer, Seivewright, Ferguson, Murphy, and Johnson	1993	181 patients with GAD, PD, or dysthymia	Pharmacotherapy, cognitive therapy, or self-help.	The presence of a personality disorder was associated with a poorer outcome of CBT and self–help at 2-year follow-up.	
Seivewright, Tyrer, and Johnson	1998	181 patients with GAD, PD, or dysthymia	Pharmacotherapy, cognitive therapy, or self-help.	The presence of a personality disorder predicted poorer outcome of CBT and self-help at 5-year follow-up.	
Panic disorder with and/or without agoraphobia					
Green and Curtis	1988	25 patients with PD/A (13 had at least one personality disorder)	Pharmacological treatment (alprazolam, imipramine, or placebo)	The presence of one or more personality disorder, and the presence of AVPD were associated wih relapse.	
Reich	1988	52 patients with PD/A (19 had at least one personality disorder)	Pharmacological treatment (alprazolam or diazepam)	The presence of antisocial, borderline, narcissistic, and histrionic personality disorders was associated with poorer outcomes on all measures, except for spontaneous panic attacks.	
Marchand and Wapler	1993	41 patients with PDA	CBT	No differences were found on outcome with regard to the presence or absence of a personality disorder.	
Keijsers, Schaap, and Hoogduin	1994	60 patients with PD/A	Behavioral treatment	As measured by PDQ-R scores, higher personality psychopathology was associated with higher levels of agoraphobic avoidance and higher frequency of panic attacks at posttest.	The relationship was no longer significant after adjusting for multiple tests.
Dreessen, Arntz, Luttels, and Sallaerts	1994 (1st study)	31 patients with PD/A (14 had at least one personality disorder)	CBT	No influence on outcome was found with regard to the presence of a personality disorder.	OCPD traits predicted worse outcome at posttest, 1-month, and 6-month follow-up. Borderline personality traits predicted better outcome at 6-month follow-up.

Authors	Year	Participants	Treatment	Influence of personality disorders on outcome	Other results
Black et al.	1994	66 patients with PD/A (23 had at least one personality disorder when measured by SIDP-R, and 22 had at least one personality disorder when measured by PDQ)	Cognitive therapy, pharmacotherapy, or placebo.	The presence of a personality disorder was not a predictor of treatment outcome at week 4, when personality was assessed by the SIDP-R.	The presence of a personality disorder was a negative predictor of outcome at week 4 in groups receiving cognitive therapy or placebo, when personality was assessed by a self-report questionnaire (PDQ).
Fava et al.	1995	110 patients with PDA	Behavioral treatment	The presence of a personality disorder was associated with a decreased likelihood of remission for 7 years after treatment.	
Rathus, Sanderson, Miller, and Wetzler	1995	18 patients with PDA (10 had at least one personality disorder)	CBT	No differences were found on outcome measures with regard to the presence or absence of a personality disorder.	
Hofmann et al.	1998	93 patients with PD/A	CBT or pharmacotherapy	Personality disorder traits did not predict outcome of treatments.	
Chambless et al.	2000	49 patients with PDA (27% had AVPD)	Behavioral treatment	AVPD predicted less improvement in the frequency of panic attacks at the 6-month follow-up.	
Toni et al.	2000	326 patients with PD/A	Pharmacological treatment (antidepressants, mainly imipramine, clomipramine, and paroxetine)	Personality disorders were not associated with outcome of treatment.	
Berger et al.	2004	73 patients with PD/A (23 had at least one personality disorder)	Pharmacological treatment (paroxetine) or pharmacological treatment + cognitive therapy	The presence of a personality disorder, particularly AVPD, was associated with poorer response to treatment.	
Prasko et al.	2005	60 patients with PD/A (29 had at least one personality disorder)	Pharmacological treatment (SSRI) + CBT (15 patients received CBT only)	The presence of a personality disorder was associated with poorer outcomes on most measures.	There were no differences on overall symptoms of anxiety, with regard to the presence or absence of a personality disorder.

Authors	Year	Participants	Treatment	Influence of personality disorders on outcome	Other results
Marchesi et al.	2006	71 patients with PD/A (38 had at least one personality disorder)	Pharmacological treatment (paroxetine or citalopram)	BPD traits were negatively associated with remission of panic attacks	
Kampman, Keijsers, Hoogduin, and Hendriks	2008	161 patients with PD/A (of the 129 completers, 60 had at least one Cluster C personality disorder, and 47 had AVPD)	CBT	The presence of Cluster C personality disorders was not associated with outcome of treatment.	
Telch, Kamphuis, and Schmidt	2011	173 patients with PD/A (54 had at least one personality disorder)	CBT	The presence of one or more personality disorders was associated with a poorer outcome of CBT at posttest, when baseline severity of panic disorder was not controlled.	When baseline severity was controlled, Cluster A and C personality disorders were associated with poorer outcome. When assessed dimensionally, only Cluster C traits were associated with poorer outcome.
Obsessive-compulsive disorder					
Jenike, Baer, Minichiello, Schwartz, and Carey	1986	43 patients with OCD (14 with a schizotypal personality disorder and 29 without a schizotypal personality disorder)	Pharmacotherapy, Behavior therapy, or a combination of both	The presence of a schizotypal personality disorder predicted poorer response to both types of treatment.	
Minichiello, Baer, and Jenike	1987	29 patients with OCD (10 with a schizotypal personality disorder and 19 without a schizotypal personality disorder)	Behavioral treatment or Behavioral treatment + Pharmacological treatment	The presence of a schizotypal personality disorder was negatively associated with outcome.	The number of schizotypal traits was also negatively associated with outcome.
Steketee	1990	26 patients with OCD (13 had at least one	Behavioral treatment	Personality disorders were not associated with treatment outcome.	Dependent and avoidant traits were

Authors	Year	Participants	Treatment	Influence of personality disorders on outcome	Other results
		personality disorder)			associated with better outcomes.
Baer and Jenike	1990	67 patients with OCD	Pharmacological treatment (fluoxetine)	The presence of an AVPD was associated with more improvement on OCD symptoms.	
Baer et al.	1992	55 patients with OCD (33 had at least one personality disorder)	Pharmacological treatment (clomipramine)	The presence of schizotypal personality disorder, AVPD, and BPD was associated with poorer outcomes.	The presence of any Cluster A diagnosis, and the number of personality disorders diagnosed were associated with poorer outcomes.
Maina, Bellino, and Bogetto	1993	48 patients with OCD (44 had at least one personality disorder)	Pharmacological treatment	Number of personality disorders diagnosed, and the presence of a schizotypal personality disorder were associated with chronicity of OCD	
Ravizza, Barzega, Bellino, Bogetto, and Maina	1995	53 patients with OCD (28% (n=15) had a schizotypal personality disorder)	Pharmacological treatment (clomipramine or fluoxetine)	The presence of a schizotypal personality disorder was associated with nonresponse to treatment.	
Cavedini, Erzegovesi, Ronchi, and Bellodi	1997	30 patients with OCD (9 with an OCPD and 21 without an OCPD)	Pharmacological treatment (clomipramine or fluvoxamine)	The presence of an OCPD predicted poorer treatment outcome.	
Dreessen, Hoekstra, and Arntz	1997	52 patients with OCD (of the 43 completers, 22 had at least one personality disorder)	Behavior therapy, Cognitive therapy, or CBT	Personality disorders were not associated with outcome of treatment.	
Fricke et al.	2005	55 patients with OCD (24 had at least one personality disorder)	CBT	The presence of a personality disorder was not associated with treatment outcome.	
Hansen, Vogel, Stiles, and Götestam	2007	35 patients with OCD (24 had at least one personality disorder)	CBT or Behavior therapy + relaxation training	The presence of Cluster A or B personality disorders was associated with poorer outcomes at 12-month follow-up, in both treatment conditions.	

Authors	Year	Participants	Treatment	Influence of personality disorders on outcome	Other results
Generalized anxiety disorder					
Mancuso, Townsend, and Mercante	1993	44 patients with GAD	Pharmacological treatment (adinazolam or placebo)	The presence of a personality disorder, particularly in Cluster B or C, was negatively associated with remission 16 months after treatment.	
Sanderson, Beck, and McGinn	1994	22 patients with GAD (9 had at least one personality disorder)	Cognitive therapy	Personality disorders were not associated with treatment outcome.	Patients with personality disorders were more likely to drop out of treatment.
Social phobia					
Turner	1987	13 patients with social phobia (7 had at least one personality disorder)	CBT	Patients with personality disorders improved less on most outcome measures during treatment.	
Mersch, Jansen, and Arntz	1995	34 patients with social phobia (8 had at least one personality disorder)	Behavioral treatment or CBT	Personality disorders did not influence the outcome of treatment.	
Hofmann, Newman, Becker, Taylor, and Roth	1995	16 patients with social phobia (8 with an AVPD and 8 without an AVPD)	Behavioral treatment	Patients with and without an AVPD improved as much with treatment.	
Brown, Heimberg, and Juster	1995	102 patients with social phobia (28 with an AVPD and 74 without an AVPD)	CBT	The presence of an AVPD did not predict treatment outcome.	
Hope, Herbert, and White	1995	23 patients with social phobia (14 with an AVPD and 9 without an AVPD)	CBT	The presence of an AVPD did not predict treatment outcome.	
Feske, Perry, Chambless, Renneberg, and Goldstein	1996	48 patients with generalized social phobia (35 with an AVPD and 13 without an AVPD)	Behavioral treatment	The presence of an AVPD was associated with less improvement on trait anxiety and self-esteem during treatment, but no differences were found with regard to depression,	However, patients with an AVPD continued to be more severely impaired at posttest and follow-up. When baseline depression was

Authors	Year	Participants	Treatment	Influence of personality disorders on outcome	Other results
				social adjustment and social phobic complaints. Patients with and without an AVPD improved at the same rate during the follow-up period.	controlled, AVPD no longer predicted improvement during treatment.
Versiani et al.	1996	101 patients with social phobia	Pharmacological treatment (moclobemide)	Personality disorders predicted nonresponse to treatment.	
Van Velzen, Emmelkamp, and Scholing	1997	61 patients with social phobia (30 without any personality disorder, 18 with an AVPD, and 13 with multiple personality disorders)	Behavioral treatment	Personality disorders did not influence the outcome of treatment.	
Posttraumatic stress disorder					
Feeny, Zoellner, and Foa	2002	72 women with PTSD (7 with complete BPD diagnosis, 5 with partial BPD diagnosis, and 60 without a BPD)	Cognitive therapy, behavior therapy, or CBT	There were no differences between patients with and without BPD characteristics with regard to PTSD status, and measures of PTSD symptoms, anxiety and depression after treatment.	The presence of BPD characteristics was associated with a decreased likelihood of achieving good end-state functioning at posttest.
van Minnen, Arntz, and Keijsers	2002	122 patients with PTSD	Behavioral treatment	Personality disorder traits were not associated with treatment outcome, or premature termination of treatment.	
Hembree, Cahill, and Foa	2004	75 women with PTSD (29 had at least one personality disorder)	Behavioral treatment or CBT	Personality disorders did not influence the prevalence of PTSD diagnosis at posttest.	Patients with a personality disorder were less likely to achieve a good end-sate functioning after treatment.
Clarke, Rizvi, and Resick	2008	131 women with PTSD	Cognitive therapy or behavior therapy	Patients with higher BPD characteristics benefited as much from treatment.	

Table 1. Studies examining the influence of personality disorders on the outcome of CBT and/or pharmacological treatment for anxiety disorders

9. Mechanisms underlying the influence of personality disorders on treatment for anxiety disorders

Many arguments have been reported to explain the negative impact of personality disorders on the outcome of treatment for anxiety disorders. For instance, adverse life events have been found to be related to symptoms of anxiety and depression, and in many of those events, the individual is actively involved in both the onset and termination of the event [139]. Thus, personality disordered patients may create more negative life events for themselves, which contribute to chronic psychosocial dysfunction and increased stress [139], which in turn can negatively affect treatment outcome [32]. In addition, it has been argued that part of the differences in outcome between patients with and without personality disorders may be explained by higher drop-out rates among patients with comorbid personality disorders [32, 140]. Indeed, patients with personality disorders may experience less emotional improvement during cognitive therapy than patients without personality disorders [141]. Thus, these patients may drop out of treatment because they perceive therapy sessions as being less effective [142]. Given that compliance with treatment regimens as rated by the therapist has been associated with positive outcome of CBT for anxiety disorders [143], anxiety patients with personality pathology might comply less with treatment, which would negatively affect the outcome of intervention or lead to premature drop-out. Finally, as mentioned previously, patients with coexisting anxiety and personality disorders have been reported to have higher initial levels of symptomatology compared with anxiety patients without a personality disorder, which could account for the difference in results when baseline severity is not controlled in the analysis. When a person reports more severe symptoms at baseline, we could expect that this person would still remain more symptomatic after treatment, even though she might have improved at the same rate. In fact, the severity of symptoms before treatment has been found to predict the outcome of treatment for anxiety disorders. In one study, this baseline symptomatology has been found to be a strong predictor of end-state functioning at the 3-year follow-up test [46]. In the Telch et al. [38] study, initial levels of PD severity accounted for 27% of the explained variance in clinically significant change at posttreatment. Yet, after controlling for baseline severity of PD, results indicated that the presence of a Cluster A personality disorder still had a significant negative effect on treatment outcome, although the relationship was very modest [38].

10. Effect of treatment for anxiety disorders on personality functioning

There is evidence suggesting that treatment for Axis I disorders reduces Axis II disorders and traits. For example, Ricciardi and colleagues [144] reported that 90% of responders to OCD pharmacological and/or behavioral treatment no longer met criteria for a personality disorder, mostly avoidant, dependent, or obsessive-compulsive personality disorder. Some authors have argued that improvement of personality functioning with treatment for anxiety disorders is explained by the instruments used to assess personality, which may confound Axis I and Axis II disorders [145] or be unable to distinguish between abnormal personality traits and personality disorder symptoms [146]. Also, as mentioned previously, assessment of personality may be affected by the presence of Axis I disorders, which would explain improvement in personality functioning with improvement of OCD symptoms [144]. In addition, three studies [147-149] have found a reduction of avoidant personality traits after pharmacological treatment for social phobia. However, most of the studies that examined changes in personality functioning with anxiety disorder treatment were conducted among patients with PD. Thus, improvement in personality functioning with cognitive and/or behavioral treatment for PD has been demonstrated more than once [61, 62, 146, 150, 151]. For instance, PD patients treated with CBT have been reported to show significant decline in all personality disorder subscales, with the exception of schizoide personality traits, from pretreatment to the second assessment (after the 11th session; [62]). However, the decline from the second to the third assessment (six months after the second assessment) was not significant for any of the subscales, except for the Schizoid Personality Disorder Scale, even though patients had received six additional monthly maintenance sessions during this period. Although these results were obtained when responders and nonresponders were combined, responders to CBT were found to have greater improvement in personality disorder characteristics than nonresponders to CBT [62]. In another study [150], an 82% decrease of personality disorder traits has been found among PD patients treated with cognitive therapy. Pharmacological treatment for PD has also been demonstrated to improve personality disorder characteristics [36, 62]. For example, in Marchesi et al. study [36], the rate of personality disorders has been found to decrease from 60% before treatment to 43% after treatment, and these results were mainly due to the reduction in the rate of paranoid, avoidant and dependent traits. The results obtained in these studies do not necessarily indicate that personality changes that occur after successful treatment for anxiety disorders result in a return to premorbid function [23]. Indeed, there is some evidence suggesting that these patients' personalities still remain differentiable from normal controls [152]. Many suggestions have been made to explain the possible influence of anxiety disorder treatment on personality pathology. First, abnormal personality traits may be a consequence of living with an anxiety disorder [36, 61]. Thus, the personality dysfunction may decrease with the improvement of anxiety disorder symptoms. Second, an interaction or overlap of Axis I and Axis II symptoms may explain the improvement of personality dysfunction with successive treatment for Axis I disorders [20]. Third, CBT for anxiety disorders could provide general problem-solving skills to the patients, which could decrease pathological personality dysfunction [62]. In addition to the confounding assessment of personality in the presence of Axis I disorders that was reported earlier, methodological limitations may have led to these results. For example, in the Ricciardi et al. study [144], the very small sample size (n=10) may have increased the risk of type I error. Thus, we cannot exclude the possibility that their findings are only due to chance fluctuations.

11. Issues to consider in therapy

Studies have yielded conflicting conclusions regarding the influence of Axis II diagnosis on the outcome of treatment for anxiety disorders. However, anxiety patients with comorbid personality disorders were consistently reported to improve on their anxiety disorder symptoms with treatment for their anxiety disorder, even though they did not always improve as much as patients without Axis II comorbidity. Therefore, these patients should not be excluded from treatment for their anxiety disorder, because of their comorbid diagnosis [33]. Also, clinicians should be aware of their own attitude towards patients with personality disorders, given that the therapist's belief that patients with a comorbid personality disorder will not benefit from any therapy, might initiate a self fulfilling prophecy [33]. In addition, to reduce the probability of early termination of treatment among patients with comorbid personality disorders, clinicians should identify these patients early in therapy, and frequently give feedback about the therapeutic process [142]. Since most individuals with personality disorders have major issues in their interpersonal relationships, it may be difficult to establish a solid therapeutic alliance. Thus, when working with patients with dysfunctional personality, it is often necessary to monitor patients' expectation with regard to the therapeutic relationship, to be flexible in using various relationship-building techniques, to identify the inevitable "ruptures" that occur in any therapeutic context, and to work to repair such ruptures when they occur [153]. Also, the dysfunctional attitudes[1] that are central to specific personality disorders should be discussed as a first step in therapy, given that they have a functional relation to anxiety, and that the development of some ego-dystony concerning attitudes is necessary for a specific anxiety treatment to be useful [155]. Finally, when working with patients with severe personality disorders, it is recommended to use a team-based treatment approach, since it may become emotionally too difficult for an individual therapist alone to treat patients with socially disruptive behaviors, such as parasuicide, and verbal and physical aggressions [153]. Moreover, patients' interactions with several professionals could enhance the acquisition of the adaptative skills taught in therapy. Special considerations in therapy should extend to individuals who consult for their personality disorder. Indeed, when patients present a history of anxiety disorders, treatment for personality disorders should be adapted to prevent the recurrence of anxiety disorder symptoms [18].

12. Plausible explanations for conflicting results

Some of the conflicting results that were presented in this chapter may be explained by methodological flaws in the existing studies, such as low statistical power (given the small sample sizes in many studies), failure to control for baseline severity of Axis I pathology, and the use of questionnaires to assess personality dysfunction [33]. Indeed, the use of a self-report questionnaire to assess personality pathology has been criticized. Compared to interviews, self-report questionnaires would be more sensitive to state factors, such as anxiety and depression, which would lead to a higher number of personality disorder diagnosis, particularly among individuals with Axis I disorders [33]. However, results from Black and colleagues [59] are not consistent with this, given that one more patient (23 vs 22) was diag-

1 Negatively biased assumptions and beliefs regarding oneself, the world, and the future. [154]

nosed with at least one personality disorder when an interview was used to assess personality instead of a self-report questionnaire.

Furthermore, two of the studies [79, 97] reported in the Dreessen and Arntz review [33] as having yielded negative findings showed a strong trend for a higher level of personality pathology in drop-outs than in completers [32]. This may indicate that there was a negative effect of personality pathology in these studies, which was manifested in the drop-out rates [32]. Finally, the general conclusions drawn from the Dreessen and Arntz review [33] should be carefully interpreted. Indeed, some studies were reported as having no effect of personality on outcome, although when examined separately, there was at least a moderate effect [32]. As mentioned by Reich [32], it was reported in the review that Dreessen and colleagues [58] obtained negative results, although obsessive-compulsive personality traits were related negatively to treatment outcome, and they reported negative findings for the Black et al. [59] study when it was actually concluded that the presence of a personality disorder was a predictor of poor outcome in the non SSRI-treated group when the self-report questionnaire was used to assess personality pathology.

13. Future area of research

Even though studies have yielded conflicting conclusions regarding the influence of Axis II diagnosis on the outcome of treatment for anxiety disorders, most studies examining the outcome of treatment for PD and OCD have found at least some influence of personality disorders on CBT or pharmacotherapy outcome. However, personality disorders were generally found to have no influence on the outcome of CBT for social phobia and PTSD. Yet, most studies on social phobia and PTSD exclusively examined the influence of specific personality disorders, AVPD and BPD, respectively, and little is known about the influence of personality disorders in general on treatment outcome for these anxiety disorders. No conclusions can be yielded from GAD studies, given that, to our knowledge, only three studies have examined the influence of personality disorders on treatment outcome for GAD, and that one of these had serious methodological limitations. Furthermore, the mechanisms that underlie the effect of Axis II disorders on the outcome of treatment for anxiety disorders are not strongly established. Future studies should concentrate on studying well reasoned hypotheses concerning these mechanisms [33] so that responsible personality variables could be understood, and intervention adapted for the needs of this specific population. For instance, the associations in course between anxiety and personality disorders may be explained by personality traits, which underlie both disorders [18], and examining these maladaptive personality traits could help us understand better the underlying mechanisms that explain the influence of personality on anxiety disorders. Although some studies have examined the influence of personality disorder traits on treatment outcome of anxiety disorders, different results have been obtained when personality was assessed dimensionally instead of categorically. In addition, improvement in the evaluation of personality is needed, to eliminate, or at least decrease, the overlap of Axis I and Axis II criteria. There is also a need for more consistency in the methods used to assess personality disorders, given that different results were obtained when personality was assessed by a self-report questionnaire instead of an interview. Further research is needed to determine whether patients with comorbid personality disorders could attain levels of posttreatment functioning equal to anxiety patients without personality dysfunction by varying duration and/or intensity of treatment sessions [38, 106], or by combining different treatment modalities [80]. Finally, more controlled prospective studies with larger sample sizes are needed to better understand the influence of personality disorders on anxiety disorders, particularly for GAD, given the small number of studies conducted among individuals with this anxiety disorder.

Author details

Véronique Palardy[1], Ghassan El-Baalbaki[1,2], Claude Bélanger[1,2] and Catherine Fredette[1]

1 University of Quebec at Montreal, Quebec, Canada

2 McGill University, Quebec, Canada

References

[1] American Psychiatric Association. Diagnostic and statistical manual of mental disorders (4th ed., text revision). Washington, DC: American Psychiatric Association; 2000.

[2] Davila J. Paths to unhappiness: The overlapping courses of depression and romantic dysfunction In: Beach SRH, editor. Marital and family processes in depression: A scientific foundation for clinical practice Washington, Dc, US: American Psychological Association 2001. p. 71-87.

[3] Ozkan M, Altindag A. Comorbid personality disorders in subjects with panic disorder: do personality disorders increase clinical severity? Comprehensive Psychiatry. 2005;46:20-6.

[4] American Psychiatric Association. DSM-V Development. Arlington, Virginia [updated May 1st, 2012]; Available from: http://www.dsm5.org/proposedrevision/Pages/PersonalityDisorders.aspx.

[5] Lenzenweger MF, Lane MC, Loranger AW, Kessler RC. DSM-IV Personality Disorders in the National Comorbidity Survey Replication. Biological psychiatry. 2007;62(6):553-64.

[6] Oldham JM, Skodol AE, Kellman HD, Hyler SE, Doidge N, Rosnick L, et al. Comorbidity of Axis I and Axis II disorders. American Journal of Psychiatry. 1995;152:571-8.

[7] Pfohl B, Black D, Noyes R, Coryell W, Barrash J. Axis I and Axis II comorbidity findings: Implications for validity In: Oldham JM, editor. Personality disorders: New per-

spectives on diagnostic validity. Washington, DC, US: American Psychiatric Association; 1991. p. 147-61.

[8] Roysamb E, Kendler KS, Tambs K, Orstavik RE, Neale MC, Aggen SH, et al. The joint structure of DSM-IV Axis I and Axis II disorders. Journal of Abnormal Psychology. 2011;120(1):198-209.

[9] Samuels J. Personality disorders: Epidemiology and public health issues. International Review of Psychiatry. 2011;23(3):223-33.

[10] Van Velzen CJM, Emmelkamp PMG. The relationship between anxiety disorders and personality disorders: Prevalance rates and comorbidity models. Treatment of personality disorders. Dordrecht, Netherlands: Kluwer Academic Publishers.; 1999. p. 129-53.

[11] Skodol AE, Oldham JM, Hyler SE, Stein DJ, Hollander E, Gallaher PE, et al. Patterns of anxiety and personality disorder comorbidity. Journal of Psychiatric Research. 1995;29(361-374).

[12] Ruegg R, Frances A. New research in personality disorders Journal of Personality Disorders. 1995;9:1-48.

[13] Dyck IR, Phillips KA, Warshaw MG, Dolan RT, Shea MT, Stout RL, et al. Patterns of Personality Pathology in Patients with Generalized Anxiety Disorder, Panic Disorder with and without Agoraphobia, and Social Phobia. Journal of Personality Disorders. 2001;15(1):60-71.

[14] Skodol AE, Gunderson JG, McGlashan TH, Dyck IR, Stout RL, Bender DS, et al. Functional impairment in patients with schizotypal, borderline, avoidant, or obsessive-compulsive personality disorder. The American Journal of Psychiatry. 2002;159(2):276-83.

[15] Johnson MR, Lydiard RB. Personality disorders in social phobia. Psychiatric Annals. 1995;25(554-563).

[16] Klass ET, Di Nardo PA, Barlow DH. DSM-III-R personality diagnoses in anxiety disorders patients. Comprehensive Psychiatry. 1989;30:251-8.

[17] Goodwin RD, Hamilton SP. Lifetime comorbidity of antisocial personality disorder and anxiety disorders among adults in the community. Psychiatry Research. 2003;117:159-66.

[18] Ansell EB, Pinto A, Edelen MO, Markowitz JC, Sanislow CA, Yen S, et al. The association of personality disorders with the prospective 7-year course of anxiety disorders. Psychological Medicine. 2011;41(5):1019-28.

[19] Shea MT, Stout RL, Yen S, Pagano ME, Skodol AE, Morey LC, et al. Associations in the Course of Personality Disorders and Axis I Disorders Over Time. Journal of Abnormal Psychology. 2004;113(4):499-508.

[20] Reich JH, Vasile RG. Effect of personality disorders on the treatment outcome of axis I conditions: An update. The Journal of Nervous and Mental Disease. 1993;181:475-84.

[21] Johnson JG, Cohen P, Kasen S, Brooks JS. Personality disorders evident by early adulthood and risk for anxiety disorders during middle adulthood. Journal of Anxiety Disorders. 2006;20:408-26.

[22] Bachar E, Hadar H, Shalev A, Y. Narcissistic vulnerability and the development of PTSD: A prospective study. Journal of Nervous and Mental Disease. 2005;193:762-5.

[23] Brandes M, Bienvenu OJ. Anxiety disorders and personality disorders comorbidity. In: Stein MB, Antony MM, editor. Oxford handbook of anxiety and related disorders. Oxford: Oxford University Press; 2009. p. 587-95.

[24] Widiger TA, Shea MT. The differentiation of Axis I and Axis II disorders. Journal of Abnormal Psychology. 1991;100:399-406.

[25] Reich J. Avoidant and dependent personality traits in relatives of patients with panic disorder, patients with dependent personality disorder, and normal controls. Psychiatry Research. 1991;39:89-98.

[26] Samuels J, Nestadt G, Bienvenu OJ, Costa PTJ, Riddle MA, Liang KY, et al. Personality disorders and normal personality dimensions in obsessive-compulsive disorder. British Journal of Psychiatry. 2000;177:457-62.

[27] Dolan-Sewell RT, Krueger RF, Shea MT. Co-occurrence with syndrome disorders. In: Livesley WJ, editor. Handbook of personality disorders. New York: Guilford Press; 2001. p. 84-104.

[28] Lewinsohn PM, Rohde P, Seeley JR, Klein DN. Axis II psychopathology as a function of Axis I disorders in childhood and adolescence. Journal of the American Academy of Child and Adolescent Psychiatry. 1997;36:1752-9.

[29] Kasen S, Cohen P, Skodol A, E., Johnson JG, Smailes E, Brooks JS. Childhood depression and adult personality disorder: Alternative pathways of continuity. Archives of General Psychiatry. 2001;58:231-6.

[30] Mennin DS, Heimberg RG. The impact of comorbid mood and personality disorders in the cognitive-behavioral treatment of panic disorder. Clinical Psychology Review. 2000;20(3):339-57.

[31] Reich JH, Green AI. Effect of personality disorders on outcome of treatment. The Journal of Nervous and Mental Disease. 1991;179:74-82.

[32] Reich J. The effect of Axis II disorders on the outcome of treatment of anxiety and unipolar depressive disorders: A review Journal of Personality Disorders. 2003;17(5): 387-405.

[33] Dreessen L, Arntz A. The impact of personality disorders on treatment outcome of anxiety disorders: Best-evidence synthesis. Behaviour Research and Therapy. 1998;36:483-504.

[34] Chambless DL, Renneberg B, Goldstein A, Gracely E. MCMI-diagnosed personality disorders among agoraphobic outpatients: Prevalence and relationship to severity and treatment outcome. Journal of Anxiety Disorders. 1992;6:193-213.

[35] Green MA, Curtis GC. Personality disorders in panic patients: Response to termination of treatment. Journal of Personality Disorders. 1988;2:303-14.

[36] Marchesi C, Cantoni A, Fontò S, Giannelli MR, Maggini C. The effect of pharmacotherapy on personality disorders in panic disorder: A one year naturalistic study. Journal of Affective Disorders. 2005;89((1-3)):189-94.

[37] Mellman TA, Leverich GS, Hauser P, Kramlinger K, Post RM, Uhde TW. Axis II pathology in panic and affective disorders: Relationship to diagnosis, course of illness, and treatment response. Journal of Personality Disorders. 1992;6:53-63.

[38] Telch MJ, Kamphuis JH, Schmidt NB. The effects of comorbid personality disorders on cognitive behavioral treatment for panic disorder. Journal of Psychiatric Research. 2011;45(4):469-74.

[39] Tyrer P, Gunderson J, Lyons M, Tohen M. Special feature: Extent of comorbidity between mental state and personality disorders. Journal of Personality Disorders. 1997;11:242-59.

[40] Friedman CJ, Shear MK, Frances AJ. DSM-III personality disorders in panic patients. Journal of Personality Disorders. 1987;1(2):132-5.

[41] Pollack MH, Otto MW, Rosenbaum JF, Sachs GS. Personality disorders in patients with panic disorder: Association with childhood anxiety disorders, early trauma, comorbidity, and chronicity. Comprehensive Psychiatry. 1992;33(2):78-83.

[42] Reich JH. DSM-III personality disorders and the outcome of treated panic disorder. American Journal of Psychiatry. 1988;145:1149-52.

[43] Marchand A, Goyer LR, Dupuis G, Mainguy N. Personality disorders and the outcome of cognitive, behavioural treatment of panic disorder with agoraphobia. Canadian Journal of Behavioural Science/Revue canadienne des sciences du comportement. 1998;30(1):14-23.

[44] Dammen T, Ekeberg O, Arnesen H, Friis S. Personality profiles in patients referred for chest pain: Investigation with emphasis on panic disorder patients. Psychosomatics. 2000;41:269-76.

[45] Mavissakalian M, Hamann MS, Jones B. A comparison of DSM-III personality disorders in panic/agoraphobia and obsessive-compulsive disorder. Comprehensive Psychiatry. 1990;31(3):238-44.

[46] Noyes R, Reich J, Christiansen J, Suelzer M, Pfohl B, Coryell WA. Outcome of panic disorder: Relationship to diagnostic subtypes and comorbidity. Archives of General Psychiatry. 1990;47:809-18.

[47] Alnaes R, Torgersen S. A 6-year follow-up study of anxiety disorders in psychiatric outpatients : development and continuity with personality disorders and personality traits as predictors. Nordic Journal of Psychiatry. 1999;53:409-16.

[48] Friedman S, Jones JC, Chernen L, Barlow DH. Suicidal ideation and suicide attempts among patients with panic disorder: a survey of two outpatient clinics. American Journal of Psychiatry. 1992;149:680-5.

[49] Iketani T, Kiriike N, Stein MB, Nagao K, Minamikawa N, Shidao A, et al. Patterns of axis II comorbidity in early-onset versus late-onset of panic disorder in Japan. Comprehensive Psychiatry. 2004;45:114-20.

[50] Starcevic V, Bogojevic G, Marinkovic J, Kelin K. Axis I and Axis II comorbidity in panic/agoraphobic patients with and without suicidal ideation. Psychiatry Research. 1999;88:153-61.

[51] Mavissakalian M, Hamann MS. DSM-III personality disorders in agoraphobia. Comprehensive Psychiatry. 1986;27:471-9.

[52] Tyrer P, Seivewright N, Ferguson B, Murphy S, Johnson LA. The Nottingham study of neurotic disorder: Effect of personality status on response to drug treatment, cognitive therapy and self help over two years. British Journal of Psychiatry. 1993;162:219-26.

[53] Seivewright N, Tyrer P, Johnson T. Prediction of outcome in neurotic disorder: A 5 year prospective study. Psychological Medicine. 1998;28:1149-57.

[54] Fava GA, Zielezny M, Savron G, Grandi S. Long-term effects of behavioural treatment for panic disorder with agoraphobia. British Journal of Psychiatry. 1995;166(1): 87-92.

[55] Keijsers GPJ, Schaap CPDR, Hoogduin CAL. Prognostic factors in the behavioral treatment of panic disorder with and without agoraphobia Behavior Therapy. 1994; 25:689-708.

[56] Hyler SE, Skodol AE, Kellman HD, Oldham JM, et al. Validity of the Personality Diagnostic Questionnaire-Revised: Comparison with two structured interviews. The American Journal of Psychiatry. 1990;147(8):1043-8.

[57] Chambless DL, Renneberg B, Gracely EJ, Goldstein AJ, Fydrich T. Axis I and II comorbidity in agoraphobia: prediction of psychotherapy outcome in a clinical setting. Psychotherapy Research. 2000;10(3):279-95.

[58] Dreessen L, Arntz A, Luttels C, Sallaerts S. Personality disorders do not influence the results of cognitive behavior therapies for anxiety disorders. Comprehensive Psychiatry. 1994;35(265-274).

[59] Black DW, Wesner RB, Gabel J, Bowers W, Monahan P. Predictors of short-term treatment response in 66 patients with panic disorder. Journal of Affective Disorders. 1994;30:233-41.

[60] Marchand A, Wapler M. L'effet des troubles de personnalite sur la reponse au traitement behavioral-cognitif du trouble panique avec agoraphobie. Revue Canadienne de Psychiatrie. 1993;38:163-6.

[61] Rathus J, Sanderson WC, Miller AL, Wetzler S. Impact of personality functioning on cognitive behavioral therapy of panic disorder: A preliminary report. Journal of Personality Disorders. 1995;9:160-8.

[62] Hofmann SG, Shear MK, Barlow DH, Gorman JM, Hershberger D, Patterson M, et al. Effects of panic disorder treatments on personality disorder characteristics. Depression and Anxiety. 1998;8:14-20.

[63] Klein MH, Benjamin LS, Rosenfeld R, Treece C, Husted J, Greist JH. The Wisconsin Personality Disorders Inventory: Development, Reliability, and Validity. Journal of Personality Disorders. 1993;7(4):285-303.

[64] Kampman M, Keijsers GPJ, Hoogduin CAL, Hendriks G-J. Outcome prediction of cognitive behaviour therapy for panic disorder: initial symptom severity is predictive for treatment outcome, comorbid anxiety or depressive disorder, cluster C personality disorders and initial motivation are not. Behavioural and Cognitive Psychotherapy. 2008;36:99-112.

[65] Hyler SE, Skodol AE, Oldham JM, Kellman HD, Doidge N. Validity of the Personality Diagnostic Questionnaire-Revised: a replication in an outpatient sample. Comprehensive Psychiatry. 1992;33:73-7.

[66] Slaap BR, den Boer JA. The prediction of nonresponse to pharmacotherapy in panic disoder: a review. Depression and Anxiety. 2001;14:112-22.

[67] Marchesi C, De Panfilis C, Cantoni A, Fontò S, Giannelli MR, Maggini C. Personality disorders and response to medication treatment in panic disorder: A 1-year naturalistic study. Progress in Neuro-Psychopharmacology & Biological Psychiatry 2006;30(7):1240-5.

[68] Toni C, Perugi G, Frare F, Mata B, Vitale B, Mengali F, et al. A prospective naturalistic study of 326 panic-agoraphobic patients treated with antidepressants. Pharmacopsychiatry. 2000;33:121-31.

[69] Berger P, Sachs G, Amering M, Holzinger A, Bankier B, Katschnig H. Personality disorder and social anxiety predict delayed response in drug and behavioral treatment of panic disorder. Journal of Affective Disorders. 2004;80:75-8.

[70] Prasko J, Houbova P, Novak T, Zalesky R, Espa-Cervena K, Paskova B, et al. Influence of personality disorders on the treatment of panic disorder- comparison study. Neuro Endocrinology Letters. 2005;26:667-74.

[71] Hamilton M. The assessment of anxiety states by rating. British Journal of Medical Psychology. 1959;32(1):50-5.

[72] Beck AT, Epstein N, Brown G, Steer RA. An inventory for measuring clinical anxiety: Psychometric properties. Journal of Consulting and Clinical Psychology 1988;56:893-7.

[73] Bejerot S, Ekselius L, von Knorring L. Comorbidity between obsessive-compulsive disorder (OCD) and personality disorders. Acta Psychiatrica Scandinavica. 1998;97:398-402.

[74] Cao W-S, Yu H-H, Jiao Z-A. Comorbidity of obsessive-compulsive disorder with personality disorders. Chinese Mental Health Journal. 2011;25(2):98-101.

[75] Horesh N, Dolberg OT, Kirschenbaum Aviner N, Kotler M. Personality differences between obsessive-compulsive disorder subtypes: Washers versus checkers. Psychiatry Research. 1997;71:197-200.

[76] Matsunaga H, Kiriike N, Miyata A, al. e. Personality disorders in patients with obsessive-compulsive disorder in Japan. Acta Psychiatrica Scandinavica. 1998;98:128-34.

[77] Steketee G. Personality traits and disorders in obsessive-compulsives. Journal of Anxiety Disorders. 1990;4:351-64.

[78] Cavedini P, Erzegovesi S, Ronchi P, Bellodi L. Predictive value of obsessive-compulsive personality disorder in antiobsessional pharmacological treatment. European Neuropsychopharmacology. 1997;7:45-9.

[79] Dreessen L, Hoekstra R, Arntz A. The influence of personality disorders on cognitive behavioral therapy for obsessive compulsive disorder. Journal of Anxiety Disorders. 1997;11:503-21.

[80] Fricke S, Moritz S, Andresen B, Jacobsen D, Kloss M, Rufer M, et al. Do personality disorders predict negative treatment outcome in obsessive-compulsive dsorders? A prospective 6-month follow-up study. European Psychiatry. 2005;21:319-24.

[81] Tenney NH, Schotte CK, Denys DA, van Megen HJ, Westenberg HG. Assessment of DSM-IV personality disorders in obsessive-compulsive disorder: Comparison of clinical diagnosis, self-report questionnaire, and semi-structured interview. Journal of Personality Disorders. 2003;17:550-61.

[82] Bogetto F, Barzega G, Bellino S, Maina G, Ravizza L. Obsessive-compulsive disorder and personality dimension: A study report. European Journal of Psychiatry. 1997;11:156-61.

[83] Baer L, Jenike MA, Ricciardi JN, Holland AD, et al. Standardized assessment of personality disorders in obsessive-compulsive disorder. Archives of General Psychiatry. 1990;47(9):826-30.

[84] Joffe RT, Swinson RP, Regan JJ. Personality features in obsessive-compulsive disorder. American Journal of Psychiatry. 1988;145:1127-9.

[85] Maina G, Albert U, Salvi V, Pessina E, Bogetto F. Early-onset obsessive-compulsive disorder and personality disorders in adulthood. Psychiatry Research. 2008;158:217-25.

[86] Baer L, Jenike A. Personality disorders in obsessive compulsive disorder. Psychiatric Clinics of North America. 1992;15:803-12.

[87] Jenike MA, Baer L, Minichiello WE, Schwartz CE, Carey JRJ. Concomitant obsessive–compulsive disorder and schizotypal personality disorder. American Journal of Psychiatry. 1986;143(4):530-2.

[88] Minichiello WE, Baer L, Jenike MA. Schizotypal personality disorder: a poor prognostic indicator for behavior therapy in the treatment of obsessive–compulsive disorder. Journal of Anxiety Disorders. 1987;1:273-6.

[89] Moritz S, Fricke S, Jacobsen D, Kloss M, Wein C, Rufer M, et al. Positive schizotypal symptoms predict treatment outcome in obsessive-compulsive disorder. Behaviour Research and Therapy. 2004;42:217-27.

[90] Ravizza L, Barzega G, Bellino S, Bogetto F, Maina G. Predictors of drug treatment response in obsessive–compulsive disorder. Journal of Clinical Psychiatry. 1995;56(8): 368-73.

[91] Hansen B, Vogel PA, Stiles TC, Götestam KG. Influence of co-morbid generalized anxiety disorder, panic disorder and personality disorders on the outcome of cognitive behavioural treatment of obsessive-compulsive disorder. Cognitive Behaviour Therapy. 2007;36(3):145-55.

[92] Maina G, Bellino S, Bogetto F, Ravizza L. Personality disorders in obsessive-compulsive patients: a study report. The European Journal of Psychiatry. 1993;7:155-63.

[93] Baer L, Jenike MA, Black DW, Treece C, Rosenfeld R, Greist J. Effect of Axis II diagnoses on treatment outcome with clomipramine in 55 patients with obsessive–compulsive disorder. Archives of General Psychiatry. 1992;49(11):862-6.

[94] Baer L, Jenike MA. Personality Disorders in Obsessive–Compulsive Disorder. In: Jenike MA, Baer L, Minichiello WE, editor. Obsessive–Compulsive Disorders: Theory and Management: Year Book Medical Publishers, Inc.; 1990.

[95] Massion AO, Dyck IR, Shea MT, Phillips KA, Warshaw MG, Keller MB. Personality disorders and time to remission in generalized anxiety disorder, social phobia, and panic disorder. Archives of General Psychiatry. 2002;59:434-40.

[96] Mauri M, Sarno N, Rossi VM, Armani A, Zambotto S, Cassano GB, et al. Personality disorders associated with generalized anxiety, panic, and recurrent depressive disorders. Journal of Personality Disorders. 1992;6:162-7.

[97] Sanderson WC, Beck AT, McGinn LK. Cognitive therapy for generalized anxiety disorder: Significance of comorbid personality disorders. Journal of Cognitive Psychotherapy. 1994;8(1):13-8.

[98] Sanderson WC, Wetzler S, Beck AT, Betz F. Prevalence of personality disorders in patients with anxiety disorders. Psychiatry Research. 1994;51:167-74.

[99] Blashfield R, Noyes R, Reich J, Woodman C, B. C, Garvey M. Personality disorder traits in generalized anxiety and panic disorder patients. Comprehensive Psychiatry. 1994;35(329-334).

[100] Gasperini M, Battaglia M, Diaferia G, Balladi L. Personality features related to generalized anxiety disorder. Comprehensive Psychiatry. 1990;31(4):363-8.

[101] Nesdadt MB, Romanoski AJ, Samuels JF, Folstein MF, McHugh PR. The relationship between personality and DSM-III axis I disorders in the population: results from an epidemiologic survey. American Journal of Psychiatry. 1992;149:1228-33.

[102] Mancuso DM, Townsend MH, Mercante DE. Long-term follow-up of generalized anxiety disorder. Comprehensive Psychiatry. 1993;34:441-6.

[103] Reich J, Perry JC, Shera D, Dyck I, et al. Comparison of personality disorders in different anxiety disorder diagnoses: Panic, agoraphobia, generalized anxiety, and social phobia. Annals of Clinical Psychiatry. 1994;6(2):125-34.

[104] Sanderson WC, Barlow DH. A description of patients diagnosed with DSM-III-R generalized anxiety disorder. Journal of Nervous and Mental Disease. 1990;178:588-91.

[105] Jansen MA, Arntz A, Merckelbach H, Mersch PPA. Personality disorders and features in social phobia and panic disorder. Journal of Abnormal Psychology. 1994;103(2):391-5.

[106] Mersch PPA, Jansen MA, Arntz A. Social phobia and personality disorder: Severity of complaint and treatment effectiveness. Journal of Personality Disorders. 1995;9:143-59.

[107] Turner SM, Beidel DC, Borden JW, Stanley MA, Jacob RG. Social phobia: Axis I and II correlates. Journal of Abnormal Psychology. 1991;100(1):102-6.

[108] Bienvenu OJ, Stein MB. Personality and anxiety disorders: a review. Journal of Personality Disorders. 2003;17(2):139-51.

[109] Brooks RB, Baltazar PL, Munjack DJ. Co-occurrence of personality disorders with panic disorder, social phobia, and generalized anxiety disorder: A review of the literature. Journal of Anxiety Disorders. 1989;3(4):259-85.

[110] Van Velzen CJM, Emmelkamp PMG, Scholing A. The impact of personality disorders on behavioral treatment outcome for social phobia. Behaviour Research and Therapy. 1997;35:889-900.

[111] Feske U, Perry KJ, Chambless DL, Renneberg B, Goldstein AJ. Avoidant personality disorder as a predictor for treatment outcome among generalized social phobics. Journal of Personality Disorders. 1996;10:174-84.

[112] Herbert JD, Hope DA, Bellack AS. Validity of the distinction between generalized social phobia and avoidant personality disorder. Journal of Abnormal Psychology. 1992;101:332-9.

[113] Hofmann SG, Newman MG, Becker E, Taylor CB, Roth WT. Social phobia with and without avoidant personality disorder: Preliminary behavior therapy outcome findings. Journal of Anxiety Disorders. 1995;2:427-38.

[114] Schneier FR, Spitzer RL, Gibbon M, Fyer AJ, Liebowitz MR. The relationship of social phobia subtypes and avoidant personality disorder. Comprehensive Psychiatry. 1991;32:496-502.

[115] Reich J. The relationship of social phobia to avoidant personality disorder: a proposal to reclassify avoidant personality disorder based on clinical empirical findings European Psychiatry. 2000;15:151-9.

[116] Widiger TA. Generalized social phobia versus avoidant personality disorder: A commentary on three studies. Journal of Abnormal Psychology. 1992;101:340-3.

[117] Reichborn-Kjennerud T, Czajkowski N, Torgersen S, Neale MC, Ørstavik RE, Tambs K, et al. The Relationship Between Avoidant Personality Disorder and Social Phobia: A Population-Based Twin Study. American Journal of Psychiatry. 2007;164:1722-8.

[118] Brown EJ, Heimberg RG, Juster HR. Social phobia subtype and avoidant personality disorder: Effect on severity of social phobia, impairment, and outcome of cognitive behavioral treatment. Behavior Therapy. 1995;26(467-486).

[119] Hope DA, Herbert JD, White C. Diagnostic subtype, avoidant personality disorder, and efficacy of cognitive-behavioral group therapy for social phobia. Cognitive Therapy and Research. 1995;19:399-417.

[120] Turner RM. The effects of personality disorder diagnosis on the outcome of social anxiety symptom reduction. Journal of Personality Disorders. 1987;1:136-43.

[121] Versiani M, Nardi AE, Mindim FD, Pinto S, Saboya E, Kovacs R. The long-term treatment of social phobia with moclobemide. International Clinical Psychopharmacology. 1996;11 ((suppl 3)):83-8.

[122] Faustman WO, White PA. Diagnostic and psychopharmacological treatment characteristics of 536 inpatients with posttraumatic stress disorder. Journal of Nervous and Mental Disease. 1989;177(3):154-9.

[123] Southwick SM, Yehuda R, Giller EL. Personality disorders in treatment seeking combat veterans with posttraumatic stress disorder. American Journal of Psychiatry. 1993;150:1020-3.

[124] Shea MT, Zlotnick C, Weisberg RB. Commonality and specificity of personality disorder profiles in subjects with trauma histories. Journal of Personality disorders. 1999;13:199-210.

[125] Dunn NJ, Yanasak E, Schillaci J, Simotas S, Rehm LP, Souchek J, et al. Personality Disorders in Veterans With Posttraumatic Stress Disorder and Depression. Journal of Traumatic Stress. 2004;17(1):75-82.

[126] Hembree EA, Cahill SP, Foa EB. Impact of Personality Disorders on Treatment Outcome for Female Assault Survivors with Chronic Posttraumatic Stress Disorder. Journal of Personality Disorders. 2004;18(1):117-27.

[127] Clarke SB, Rizvi SL, Resick PA. Borderline personality characteristics and treatment outcome in cognitive-behavioral treatments for PTSD in female rape victims. Behavior Therapy. 2008;39:72-8.

[128] Zlotnick C, Johnson DM, Yen S, Battle CL, Sanislow CA, Skodol A, E., et al. Clinical features and impairment in women with borderline personality disorder (BPD) with post-traumatic stress disorder (PTSD), BPD without PTSD, and other personality disorders with PTSD. Journal of Nervous and Mental Disease. 2003;191:706-13.

[129] Zanarini MC, Frankenburg FC, Dubo ED, Sickel AE, Trikha A, Levin A, et al. Axis I comorbidity of borderline personality disorder. American Journal of Psychiatry. 1998;155:1733-9.

[130] Pagura J, Stein MB, Bolton JM, Cox BJ, Grant B, Sareen J. Comorbidity of borderline personality disorder and posttraumatic stress disorder in the U.S. population. Journal of Psychiatric Research. 2010;44(16):1190-8.

[131] Ogata S, Silk K, Goodrich S, Lohr N, Westen D, Hill E. Childhood sexual and physical abuse in borderline patients. American Journal of Psychiatry. 1990;147:1008-13.

[132] Herman J, Perry J, van der Kolk B. Childhood trauma in borderline personality disorder. American Journal of Psychiatry. 1989;146(4):490-5.

[133] Goldman S, D'Angelo E, DeMaso D, Mezzacappa E. Physical and sexual abuse histories among children with borderline personality disorder. American Journal of Psychiatry. 1992;149(12):1723-6.

[134] Feeny N, Zoellner LA, Foa EB. Treatment outcome for chronic PTSD among female assaults victims with borderline personality characteristics: A preliminary examination. Journal of Personality Disorders. 2002;16:30-40.

[135] Horowitz MJ, Wilner N, Kaltreider N, Alvarez W. Signs and symptoms of posttraumatic stress disorder. Archives of General Psychiatry. 1980;37:85-92.

[136] Heffernan K, Cloitre M. A comparison of posttraumatic stress disorder with and without borderline personality disorder among women with a history of childhood sexual abuse: etiological and clinical characteristics. Journal of Nervous and Mental Disease. 2000;188(9):589-95.

[137] Zlotnick C, Franklin CL, Zimmerman M. Is comorbidity of posttraumatic stress disorder and borderline personality disorder related to greater pathology and impairment?. American Journal of Psychiatry. 2002;150:1940-3.

[138] van Minnen A, Arntz A, Keijsers GPJ. Prolonged exposure in patients with chronic PTSD: Predictors of treatment and dropout. Behaviour Research and Therapy. 2002;40:439-57.

[139] Poulton RG, Andrews G. Personality as a cause for adverse life events. Acta Psychiatrica Scandinavica. 1992;85:35-8.

[140] Grilo CM, Money R, Barlow DH, Goddard AW, Gorman JM, Hofmann SG, et al. Pretreatment patient factors predicting attrition from a multicenter randomized controlled treatment study for panic disorder. Comprehensive Psychiatry. 1998;39(323-332).

[141] Persons JB, Burns DD. Mechanisms of action of cognitive therapy: The relative contributions of technical and interpersonal interventions. Cognitive Therapy and Research. 1985;10:539-51.

[142] Persons JB, Burns DD, Perloff JM. Predictors of dropout and outcome in cognitive therapy for depression in a private practice setting. Cognitive Therapy and Research. 1988;12(6):557-75.

[143] Schmidt NB, Woolaway-Bickel K. The effects of treatment compliance on outcome in cognitive-behavioral therapy for panic disorder: quality versus quantity. Journal of Clinical Psychology. 2000;68(1):13-8.

[144] Ricciardi JN, Baer L, Jenike MA, Fischer SC, Sholtz D, Buttolph M. Changes in DSM-III-R Axis II diagnoses following treatment of Obsessive–Compulsive Disorder. American Journal of Psychiatry. 1992;149:829-31.

[145] Zimmerman M. Diagnosing personality disorders: a review of issues and research methods. Archives of General Psychiatry. 1994;51:225-45.

[146] Noyes R, Reich JH, Suelzer M, Christiansen J. Personality traits associated with panic disorder: change associated with treatment. Comprehensive Psychiatry. 1991;32(283-294).

[147] Liebowitz MR, Schneier FR, Campeas R, Hollander E, Hatterer J, Fyer A, et al. Phenelzine vs atenolol in social phobia : a placebo-controlled comparison. Archives of General Psychiatry. 1992;49:290-300.

[148] Reich J, Noyes R, Jr., Yates W. Alprazolam treatment of avoidant personality traits in social phobic patients. Journal of Clinical Psychiatry. 1989;50(91-95).

[149] Versiani M, Nardi AE, Mundim FD, Alves AB, Liebowitz MR, Amrein R. Pharmacotherapy of social phobia: A controlled study with moclobemide and phenelzine. British Journal of Psychiatry. 1992;161:353-60.

[150] Black DW, Monahan P, Wesner R, Gabel J, Bowers W. The effect of fluvoxamine, cognitive therapy, and placebo on abnormal personality traits in 44 patients with panic disorder. Journal of Personality Disorders. 1996;10:185-94.

[151] Hoffart A, Hedley LM. Personality traits among panic disorder with agoraphobia patients before and after symptom-focused treatment. Journal of Anxiety Disorders. 1997;11(1):77-87.

[152] Reich J, Noyes R, Jr., Hirschfeld R, Coryell W, O'Gorman T. State and personality in depressed and panic patients. American Journal of Psychiatry. 1987;144:181-7.

[153] Pilkonis PA. Treatment of personality disorders in association with symptom disorders In: Livesley WJ, editor. Handbook of personality disorders. New York : The Guilford Press; 2001 p. 541-54.

[154] Meyer JH, McMain S, Kennedy SH, Korman L, Brown GM, DaSilva JN, et al. Dysfunctional attitudes and 5-HT2 receptors during depression and self-harm. The American Journal of Psychiatry. 2003;160(1):90-9.

[155] Trautmann-Sponsel RD, Tominschek I, Zaudig M. Differenzielle Diagnostik und Verhaltenstherapie von Ängsten bei Persönlichkeitsstörungen. [Differential diagnosis with consequences for the behavioral therapy of anxiety in personality disorders.]. PTT: Persönlichkeitsstörungen Theorie und Therapie. 2003;7(4):211-21.

Permissions

The contributors of this book come from diverse backgrounds, making this book a truly international effort. This book will bring forth new frontiers with its revolutionizing research information and detailed analysis of the nascent developments around the world.

We would like to thank Federico Durbano, for lending his expertise to make the book truly unique. He has played a crucial role in the development of this book. Without his invaluable contribution this book wouldn't have been possible. He has made vital efforts to compile up to date information on the varied aspects of this subject to make this book a valuable addition to the collection of many professionals and students.

This book was conceptualized with the vision of imparting up-to-date information and advanced data in this field. To ensure the same, a matchless editorial board was set up. Every individual on the board went through rigorous rounds of assessment to prove their worth. After which they invested a large part of their time researching and compiling the most relevant data for our readers. Conferences and sessions were held from time to time between the editorial board and the contributing authors to present the data in the most comprehensible form. The editorial team has worked tirelessly to provide valuable and valid information to help people across the globe.

Every chapter published in this book has been scrutinized by our experts. Their significance has been extensively debated. The topics covered herein carry significant findings which will fuel the growth of the discipline. They may even be implemented as practical applications or may be referred to as a beginning point for another development. Chapters in this book were first published by InTech; hereby published with permission under the Creative Commons Attribution License or equivalent.

The editorial board has been involved in producing this book since its inception. They have spent rigorous hours researching and exploring the diverse topics which have resulted in the successful publishing of this book. They have passed on their knowledge of decades through this book. To expedite this challenging task, the publisher supported the team at every step. A small team of assistant editors was also appointed to further simplify the editing procedure and attain best results for the readers.

Our editorial team has been hand-picked from every corner of the world. Their multi-ethnicity adds dynamic inputs to the discussions which result in innovative outcomes. These outcomes are then further discussed with the researchers and contributors who give their valuable feedback and opinion regarding the same. The feedback is then collaborated with the researches and they are edited in a comprehensive manner to aid the understanding of the subject.

Apart from the editorial board, the designing team has also invested a significant amount of their time in understanding the subject and creating the most relevant covers. They scrutinized every image to scout for the most suitable representation of the subject and create an appropriate cover for the book.

The publishing team has been involved in this book since its early stages. They were actively engaged in every process, be it collecting the data, connecting with the contributors or procuring relevant information. The team has been an ardent support to the editorial, designing and production team. Their endless efforts to recruit the best for this project, has resulted in the accomplishment of this book. They are a veteran in the field of academics and their pool of knowledge is as vast as their experience in printing. Their expertise and guidance has proved useful at every step. Their uncompromising quality standards have made this book an exceptional effort. Their encouragement from time to time has been an inspiration for everyone.

The publisher and the editorial board hope that this book will prove to be a valuable piece of knowledge for researchers, students, practitioners and scholars across the globe.

List of Contributors

Ana G. Gutiérrez-García
Laboratorio de Neurofarmacología, Instituto de Neuroetología, Universidad Veracruzana, Xalapa, Veracruz, México
Facultad de Psicología, Universidad Veracruzana, Xalapa, Veracruz, México

Carlos M. Contreras
Unidad Periférica Xalapa, Instituto de Investigaciones Biomédicas, Universidad Nacional Autónoma de México, Xalapa, Veracruz, México
Laboratorio de Neurofarmacología, Instituto de Neuroetología, Universidad Veracruzana, Xalapa, Veracruz, México

John Scott Price
Retired psychiatrist, UK

Antonio Armario
Institute of Neurosciencies and Animal Physiology Unit (Department of Cellular Biology, Physiology and Immunology, School of Biosciences), Universitat Autònoma de Barcelona, Barcelona, Spain

Roser Nadal
Institute of Neurosciencies and Psychobiology Unit (Department of Psychobiology and Methodology of Health Sciences, School of Psychology), Universitat Autònoma de Barcelona, Barcelona, Spain

Meghan D. Caulfield and Richard J. Servatius
Stress & Motivated Behavior Institute, New Jersey Medical School, New Jersey, U. S. A.

Anna Boyajyan, Gohar Mkrtchyan, Lilit Hovhannisyan and Diana Avetyan
Institute of Molecular Biology, National Academy of Sciences, Yerevan, Republic of Armenia

Kevin D. Beck
Neurobehavioral Research Laboratory, Veteran Affairs New Jersey Health Care System, East Orange, NJ, USA
Stress & Motivated Behavior Institute, Department of Neurology & Neurosciences, University of Medicine & Dentistry of New Jersey - New Jersey Medical School, Newark, NJ, USA

Jennifer E. Catuzzi
University of Medicine & Dentistry of New Jersey - Graduate School of Biomedical Sciences, Newark, NJ, USA

Véronique Palardy and Catherine Fredette
University of Quebec at Montreal, Quebec, Canada

Ghassan El-Baalbaki and Claude Bélanger
McGill University, Quebec, Canada
University of Quebec at Montreal, Quebec, Canada